PSYCHED OUT

How Psychiatry Sells Mental Illness and Pushes Pills That Kill

By: Kelly Patricia O'Meara

Bloomington, IN Milton Keynes, UK

authorHOUSE™

AuthorHouse™
1663 Liberty Drive, Suite 200
Bloomington, IN 47403
www.authorhouse.com
Phone: 1-800-839-8640

AuthorHouse™ UK Ltd.
500 Avebury Boulevard
Central Milton Keynes, MK9 2BE
www.authorhouse.co.uk
Phone: 08001974150

First published by AuthorHouse 5/16/2006

ISBN: 1-4259-2662-2 (sc)
ISBN: 1-4259-2661-4 (dj)

Library of Congress Control Number: 2006902858

Printed in the United States of America
Bloomington, Indiana

This book is printed on acid-free paper.

For Margaret, Kelly, and Kevin, Jr., "Blue."
Because your clear, curious minds
are my hope for the future.

Acknowledgments

My heartfelt thanks go out to Marla Filidei and everyone at the Citizens Commission on Human Rights. During an interview six years ago Marla first made me aware of the fraud surrounding the psychiatric diagnosis ADHD. I could not have known then that this conversation would lead me into a six-year investigation into psychiatric diagnosing and mind-altering drugs, culminating in this book. Her compassion and integrity and that of the organization she represents are an example by which to live.

I am grateful to my former editors, Paul Rodriguez and Scott Stanley, at *The Washington Times'* weekly newsmagazine, *Insight on the News*. Although initially skeptical, they took a chance and gave me the go-ahead for my first article, titled *Guns & Doses*, about the connection between school shooters and psychotropic drugs. They never looked back, supporting and encouraging me to write more than two-dozen articles about the psycho-pharma debate.

A very sincere thank you to all of the dedicated men and women in the medical and scientific communities who, over the years, graciously have shared with me their experience and expertise on these issues, with a special thanks to Dr. Peter Breggin and Dr. Fred Baughman Jr., who always made themselves available to me no matter how redundant my questions might have been.

I am grateful to Cheri Seymour, Kristina Borjesson, Mary Grace and Catherine Austin Fitts for their never-ending support and encouragement. Their input, willingness to just listen and their often brutal honesty, well, these are the things that make the "count them on one hand" kind of friends.

Finally, and foremost, my unending thanks to my brother, Kevin. His love, friendship, support and encouragement truly is my greatest blessing.

Ironically, psychiatric drugs cause rather than cure biochemical imbalances in the brain. In fact, the only known biochemical imbalances in the brain of patients routinely seen by psychiatrists are brought about by the psychiatrists themselves through the prescription of mind-altering drugs. Psychiatric drugs "work" precisely by causing imbalances in the brain—by producing enough brain malfunction to dull the emotions and judgment or to produce an artificial high.
—Peter Breggin, M.D., & David Cohen, Ph.D.., *Your Drug May Be Your Problem: How and Why to Stop Taking Psychiatric Medications.*

Close to retirement at the time, Merck's aggressive chief executive, Henry Gadsden, told Fortune *magazine of his distress that the company's potential markets had been limited to sick people. Suggesting he'd rather Merck to be more like chewing gum maker Wrigley's, Gadsen said it had long been his dream to make drugs for healthy people. Because, then, Merck would be able to "sell to everyone."*
—Ray Moynihan and Alan Cassels, *Selling Sickness: How the World's Biggest Pharmaceutical Companies are Turning Us All Into Patients.*

The public at large may gain false comfort from a diagnostic psychiatric manual that encourages belief in the illusion that the harshness, brutality, and the pain in their lives and in their communities can be explained by a psychiatric label and eradicated by a pill. Certainly, there are plenty of problems that we all have and a myriad of peculiar ways that we struggle, often ineffectively, to cope with them. But could life be any different? Far too often, the psychiatric bible has been making us crazy— when we are just human.
—Herb Kutchins & Stuart A. Kirk, *Making Us Crazy: DSM: The Psychiatric Bible and the Creation of Mental Disorders.*

Author's Note

Few would argue that people suffer from mental illness, mental breakdowns, depression or any number of adjectives that describe behaviors that adversely, even severely, affect people's lives.

In law it is said that "it doesn't matter what one believes, only what one can prove." The same can be said for psychiatric diagnosing. It matters little what anyone in the medical/psychiatric community "believes" is the cause(s) of mental illness. The question that has not been answered is whether tens of millions of Americans who have been diagnosed with any one or a number of psychiatric mental disorders suffer from a mental "disease"—an objective, confirmable abnormality of the brain.

What is known is that neither the American Psychiatric Association nor the National Institute of Mental Health nor any other medical organization is capable today of making available scientific evidence to prove that any psychiatric disorder is an objective, confirmable abnormality of the brain.

This mantra is repeated throughout the book because it is the point of the book. That people are suffering isn't in question. Whether they actually suffer from a psychiatric disorder that is a known, objective, confirmable abnormality of the brain is in question because selling mental disorders as "diseases," such as the theoretical chemical imbalance, has become the norm in the medical/psycho pharmaceutical community, and it is blatantly false.

The issue is one of informed consent. In this instance—psychiatric diagnosing—the People need and deserve the whole truth. Tens of millions of Americans are daily taking dangerous mind-altering psychiatric drugs that are reported to "treat" specific alleged mental illnesses, but the pharmaceutical companies that manufacture the drugs openly admit they do not "completely" understand how the drugs work in the brain for the stated psychiatric mental disorder(s). And to top it all off, the Food and Drug Administration has determined that the psychiatric mind-altering drugs are potentially life-threatening to an unknown percentage of the population.

The People, if given the truth, can take it. The decision to accept the psychiatric diagnosis and seek treatment with psychiatric mind-

altering drugs may be no different, but at least the decision will be based on the whole truth—the objective confirmable scientific evidence—and not theories, wishful thinking, deceptive advertising or misleading advocacy group, pharmaceutical company and government-sponsored information campaigns.

To do otherwise is an injustice to the People, especially to those who are suffering and desperately looking to the medical/ scientific community for honest answers about their illness and the pharmaceutical companies for safe and effective treatment.

Important Warning:

When trying to withdraw from many psychiatric drugs, patients can develop serious and even life-threatening emotional and physical reactions. In short, it is dangerous not only to *start* taking psychiatric drugs but also can be hazardous to *stop* taking them. Therefore, withdrawal from psychiatric drugs should be done under medical and clinical supervision.

Table of Contents

Chapter One

Psychiatric Suicidal Therapy

America has a drug problem. It's nothing as covert as those illicit and illegal "Just Say No" drugs but, rather, Americans have become drug users by way of being diagnosed as suffering from one or a number of alleged mental disorders. Sharing one's feelings with a doctor more often than not is all it takes to be diagnosed with a psychiatric disorder and prescribed a mind-altering drug to "treat" the disorder.

Whether America's psychotropic drug users are "better" for having their minds chemically altered is a question that an increasing number of professionals within the medical, psychiatric and legal communities and even legislative bodies are beginning to consider. Certainly there are millions who believe prescription mind-altering drugs have made their lives more manageable and will acknowledge they feel "better" since being on psychotropic drugs. But recent revelations about Selective Serotonin Reuptake Inhibitors (SSRIs)—commonly known as antidepressants—raise serious questions about not only the effectiveness of the newest and most widely used class of psychotropic drugs, but also whether the drugs are even safe.

Whether Americans actually suffer from a biological or neurological disease (an objective, confirmable abnormality) of the brain has never been addressed by policymakers charged with ensuring the nation's mental health. That Americans are being diagnosed as mentally ill and being prescribed psychotropic drugs at startling, even epidemic rates, is not in question.

Coming up with an exact number of people currently taking prescription psychotropic drugs—which presumably would be the same number of people being diagnosed with a mental illness—is next to impossible. There is, however, scattered data from a variety of sources that provide a shocking glimpse at not only the direction the drugging of America is heading, but also the number of Americans being labeled as mentally ill.

One report claims that one in 10 women daily take antidepressants, while another study finds that in 2003 some 213 million prescriptions were written for antidepressants. Still another report claims 1.1 million new prescriptions per week were written in February 2004 alone, and yet another suggests that in 2002 nearly 11 million prescriptions for antidepressants were dispensed for children between the ages of 1 and 17. [1] The truth is there is no central clearinghouse for such information, and no single private organization or governmental body really knows how many Americans have been labeled as mentally ill and are taking prescription psychotropic drugs that are intended to alter behavior.

Graham Aldred, a citizen of Great Britain, was compelled to compile a more accurate count of persons taking the most popular SSRIs after his wife committed suicide after having been on the antidepressant Paxil, for just 11 days. Aldred's data were gathered from official sources, including the Department of Health in the United Kingdom; IMS Health, a pharmaceutical data gathering service in the United States; and the Drug Safety Research Unit (DSRU), a prescription monitoring service in Southampton, England. Aldred's model, the *IMR Patient Flow Model*, (a computer model converting medication consumed into number of patients taking drugs), analyzes the usage of the top antidepressants—Paxil, Prozac and Zoloft—in the United States since the introduction of each drug.

According to Aldred's model, Prozac, produced by Eli Lilly and Co., was introduced in the United States in 1988 and since then more than 27 million prescriptions have been written for the drug. More than 22 million Americans have been prescribed Zoloft, made by Pfizer Inc., since its introduction in 1992. Nearly 19 million Americans have been prescribed Paxil, produced by GlaxoSmithKline, since its introduction in 1993. Therefore, a grand total of nearly 68 million Americans have been prescribed and are taking at least one of the three top selling mind-altering antidepressants for behavior modification.[2]

And, while most experts believe that Aldred's model is an accurate accounting based on available data, many doctors would argue that even these numbers are conservative. There are a variety of reasons why the exact number of psychotropic drug users in the United States is unknown, the least of which involves the number of psychotropic drugs that are doled out without prescriptions as samples and, more importantly, Aldred's accounting only represents the top three of more than 30 antidepressants on the market. But researchers can say with certainty that there are, at a minimum, tens of millions of Americans—including millions of school-age children—daily taking one or several prescription mind-altering drugs. What is also certain, based on data collected by agencies of the federal government and private health-care organizations that track the trends in the use of psychotropic drugs, is that the percentage of the population labeled as mentally ill and being treated with mind-altering drugs in order to function "normally" is becoming a national health crisis.

What is less certain is the alleged benefit of psychotropic drugs prescribed for one-quarter of the U.S. population who virtually have become "users" of mind-altering drugs. Even more important is the question of whether there is science to support the psychiatric diagnosis that must be made before mind-altering drugs can be prescribed. But the record is clear on one point: Pharmaceutical companies and the psychotropic drugs they manufacture long have been blamed for the alleged harm perpetrated on the public health by antidepressants, while at the same time the psychiatric community—the doctors who create and administer the psychiatric labels that determine the public's mental health—has escaped even the most cursory of reviews. And yet it is an incontrovertible fact that the psychiatric diagnosis must precede the prescribing of psychotropic drugs.

A growing number of experts, including many psychiatrists, believe the increased use of psychotropic drugs is a two-pronged problem which, to date, has received a one-sided review by lawmakers and federal officials who set public policy. The question that remains inexplicably taboo is: Have Americans become prescription psychotropic drug users in record numbers because they suffer from objective, confirmable abnormalities of the brain?

Until the psychiatric community is called upon to provide conclusive scientific evidence that the nearly 400 disorders listed in the American Psychiatric Association's (APA's) *Diagnostic and Statistical Manual of Mental Disorders (DSM-IV)* are not merely subjective clinical diagnoses but rather objective, confirmable abnormalities of the brain, the debate surrounding the benefit or risk of psychotropic drugs seems moot. Basic logic begs the question: Without objective, confirmable proof that the neurologic-biologic abnormality exists, how can the benefit of mind-altering drug treatment be objectively determined?

While the psychiatric community thus far has succeeded in escaping any official review of the diagnoses that lead to the drugging of America, the makers of the mind-altering drugs have not been so lucky. The risk-benefit argument surrounding the use of prescription mind-altering drugs to "treat" mental disorders has been around as long as the drugs themselves. Just three short years after the 1988 U.S. introduction of Prozac (the first SSRI), the U.S. Food and Drug Administration (FDA), the federal agency tasked with oversight of the new class of antidepressant drugs, was compelled to hold public hearings to address a growing number of claims that SSRI antidepressants may harm rather than help.

The stated purpose of the 1991 FDA public hearings was "a scientific investigation into suicidal ideation, suicidal acts, and other violent behavior reported to occur in association with the pharmacological treatment of depression." In other words, the FDA was trying to determine whether this new class of mind-altering drugs was causing people to commit suicide and exhibit other violent behaviors.

It was because of "intense public interest and emotion surrounding the item on the committee's agenda" that a small number of the public that reportedly had experienced adverse reactions to the new drugs were allowed to make five-minute statements before the committee. Sally and Al Barrett explained in part their daughter's death this way: [3]

At age 17 Jennifer developed an eating disorder called anorexia. In January of 1990, however, she was placed on the antidepressant, Prozac. Several weeks later she took an overdose, which was her first suicide attempt. For the next four or five months after she was taken off this drug she did not talk about suicide nor attempt it. However, she was heavily sedated under the effects of another drug called Anafranil, and she was then placed on Prozac to counteract the effects of Anafranil. After starting Prozac, Jenny's behavior became more agitated and aggressive and hostile. Jenny started having terrorizing nightmares, frightening the whole family with her outcries. The second month after she was placed on Prozac, she secretly purchased a gun on August 25th and shot herself in the head and died on August 27th." [4]*

The committee then heard from the wife of one of the 1960's rock-and-roll recording legends, Mrs. Del Shannon. (in part)

"I am the widow of Charles Westover, also known as Del Shannon. My husband was given Prozac on January 24th of 1990. On the evening of February 8, 1990, he killed himself. I am told his death was instantaneous, but I believe his death actually began the moment he took his first dose of Prozac. Before Prozac, my husband was very involved with people, our family and his work. He was very much in charge of his business. But within days after he started taking Prozac I noticed a personality change in him.

He told me when he came home from the doctor, that he was given a new drug, 'it's not even a drug, it's a chemical, it's very safe and it's supposed to help me over the hump I'm in.' The drug was Prozac. There was absolutely no warning of suicide or anything violent. I know with absolute certainty that if Charles had any idea of the side effects of Prozac he would never have taken it. This drug is most assuredly responsible for any torment or suffering and the eventual suicide of my husband. I want people to be aware of what can happen when you take the drug Prozac." [5]

After considering all the data presented by the mental-health experts, including thousands of adverse reaction reports collected by the FDA, and listening to dozens of what can only be described as extremely compelling personal accounts of adverse reactions believed to be associated with the use of Prozac and other antidepressant drugs, by a majority vote the committee decided the data were inconclusive and voted 7-to-3 *against* recommending any additional warnings be added to the package inserts and labels of the SSRI class of antidepressants.

What the public did not know at the time of the vote by the esteemed panel of mental-health experts was that wholly one-half of the committee members had active professional and financial interests in the pharmaceutical companies that manufactured the very drugs the committee was investigating, and five of the seven votes made against a label change came from the experts with a conflict of interest. [6]

The committee's decision not to take action became a vote of confidence providing a kind of federal blessing to the pharmaceutical companies which, in the decade that followed and is now well-documented, would result in enormous increases in not only the use of SSRI antidepressants but a tenfold increase in the number of antidepressants available to the public. And with the increased use of antidepressants came an ever-increasing number of personal tragedies and horror stories believed to be associated with antidepressant use, and the public once again looked to federal regulators and policymakers for intervention.

But it wasn't until the end of 2003 when the British Committee on Safety of Medicines (CSM)—an arm of the Medicines and Healthcare products Regulatory Agency, the United Kingdom's equivalent of the FDA—effectively banned the use of seven of the top-selling antidepressants for children younger than 18 that the FDA took action. Due to an alarming number of reports of violence and self-harm in Great Britain, the British CSM beat the FDA at protecting the British citizens by conducting its own in-depth review of clinical trial data on seven of the most popular psychotropic drugs, finding that "the risk of treating depressive illness in under 18-year-olds with certain SSRIs outweigh the benefits of treatment."

There are many who believe that it was only because of the British review that the FDA finally was forced to act on numerous similar claims here in the United States. The problem, along with the drugs, had gone international and the psycho-pharmaceutical industry no longer could contain nor ignore the fact that people were not only being harmed but also that one of the most advanced Western nations had determined that the risk of taking the once reported "wonder" drugs outweighed the benefit for a growing number of the population.

Still, it's fair to say that the tens of millions of Americans daily taking a virtual smorgasbord of mind-altering antidepressants for an ever-increasing number of alleged mental disorders were clueless about the 1991 hearings, the 2003 British ban on selected antidepressants and the continuing battle in the United States, which culminated in the first of two public hearings scheduled by the FDA's Psychopharmacologic Drugs Advisory Committee and the Pediatric Subcommittee of the Anti-Infective Drugs Advisory Committee in February 2004. The stated purpose of the hearing, nearly identical to that of the 1991 hearings and the 2003 British review, was to discuss "reports of the occurrence of suicidality (both suicidal ideation and suicide attempts) in clinical trials for various antidepressant drugs in pediatric patients with major depressive disorder (MDD)." [7]

In the 13 years that followed the FDA's 1991 decision to reject warning the public of possible adverse reactions to SSRI antidepressants, the problem didn't go away. Families still believed that it was the use of the prescription mind-altering drugs that had harmed their loved ones, and it is these extraordinary personal tragedies that again led dozens of families to the Washington, D.C. area with the hope of literally getting two brief minutes before the committee to tell their unthinkable stories.

This time, when all was said and done, it was the recollections of the mothers and fathers, husbands and wives, and brothers and sisters that outweighed the data and psychobabble—including hours of jabbering about mental disorders that cannot be scientifically proven—offered by the extended panel of this nation's heavyweight mental-health experts. In the end, in so many words, the message delivered by the People was clear and concise: These drugs are killing us and we're psyched out.

Unlike other social issues, where the People are afforded the opportunity to speak to policymakers, this public hearing would break the mold. Historically, it has been the mothers who did the talking, who fight the system on behalf of the family. During this first

7

February 2004 hearing, however, a number of fathers and husbands of dead children or spouses—often choking back tears, barely able to continue—described in great detail a kind of hell that only a father or husband who feels a sense of failure, unable to protect his loved one, can know. Glenn McIntosh is one such father. With unsteady hands, McIntosh held up a photograph of his daughter for the panel of mental-health experts to see and in two minutes explained his loss and the events that he believes led to the death of his beautiful young daughter. (in part)

"I would like to introduce you to my daughter, Caitlin Elizabeth McIntosh. Well, it is actually only a two- dimensional image of her, but it is all I have left. She died of suicide at age 12 years, 3 months - just 8 weeks after being put on Paxil, and then Zoloft.

She was also having some problems sleeping due to a mild seizure disorder. We wanted to help, of course, so we took her to our family physician, who prescribed Paxil. He said it would help with her coping and her sleep. She didn't do well on it at all, so he took her off it cold turkey, which you are not supposed to do. When we saw a psychiatrist a week later, he put her on Zoloft. She then started having strong suicidal thoughts. She was put in the adolescent ward of a mental hospital to "balance her meds." Well, from there, things only got worse, as she was put on other strong psychotropic drugs to treat the symptoms that we now know were actually caused by the SSRIs. The downward spiral continued until January 5th, 2000, when she hung herself with her shoelaces in the girl's bathroom in the middle school she was attending.

We were told that antidepressants like Paxil and Zoloft were wonder drugs, that they were safe and effective for children. We were lied to. The pharmaceutical companies have known for years that these drugs could cause suicide in some patients.[8]

Mark Miller explained his son's death to the panel of mental-health experts this way: (in part)

"There is a serious problem with the way SSRI medications are being prescribed today and how, in many cases, they can directly cause violence and suicidal behavior in those we love and treasure the most—our children.

You see, we lost our 13-year-old son, Matt, in the summer of 1997. He died after a psychiatrist we did not know gave him three sample bottles of a pill we had never heard of, for a perceived illness that his doctor could only guess at. We were advised with great authority that Matt was suffering from a chemical imbalance that could be helped by a new, wonderful medication called Zoloft. It was safe, effective, only two minor side effects were cautioned with us—insomnia and indigestion. Now, I don't know if Matt had a chemical imbalance. He became agitated on the pills. He did not sleep. He did not eat. He could not sit still. That night, a Sunday, before leaving on vacation, after taking his seventh Zoloft tablet, he took his own life.[9]

Gary Cheslek spoke of his son's death from the perspective of a doctor and a father. (in part)

"My name is Gary Cheslek and my son, Justin, was a 20-year-old sophomore at the University of Southern Mississippi when he went to the Student Health Clinic complaining of insomnia. He was given a thorough examination including blood work. Significant in the doctor's note at that initial visit is the notation, 'no suicidal ideation.'

Complaining that the sleep medication he was prescribed made him feel sedated and depressed; he was put on Paxil for two weeks. During those two weeks, he repeatedly told his doctor he didn't like the way the Paxil made him feel, so he was switched to Effexor.

Within 24 hours of the switch to Effexor, he had a seizure. Five days later he hung himself in his apartment.[10]

These tragic testimonials were just a small sample of the dozens of families who seized the opportunity that frosty February day to recount similar horrific events that left them innocent victims of this new, yet undeclared "war on drugs." But only a handful of these personal tragedies were necessary before it became difficult and painfully uncomfortable to continue to listen. This was an angry, heartbroken audience and the overriding message was that physicians, psychiatrists, pharmaceutical companies and the federal agencies tasked with oversight had not been honest and had failed to make the public aware that suicidal thoughts, suicide and violent behavior were possible adverse reactions in some people who are prescribed psychiatric mind-altering antidepressants.

Perhaps the most extraordinary aspect of this February 2004 hearing was that these families, like those who went before them, could do nothing to help their own. Rather, at their own expense, both financially and emotionally, this small but committed group of families traveled to Washington in an effort to change public policy so that other parents and families would be spared from having to endure the same painful experiences. Few who spoke that day realized that they were not the first to make this trip. Few knew that they were following in the foot steps of other mothers and fathers who, more than a decade earlier, stood before the same federal agency pleading for the same protection to save other families from the same brutal heartache.

The committee's decision was too late for these and countless other families across the country grappling with the inexplicable loss of a seemingly healthy child, spouse or parent just days or weeks after beginning antidepressant treatment. But by the end of that first February 2004 hearing, the powerful players within the psycho-pharmacological community finally acted in the best interest of the People.

Although not willing to go so far as to actually connect the harmful behavior directly to the antidepressants under review, the committee acknowledged an "increased risk of suicidal thoughts and behavior [suicidality] in children and adolescents being treated with antidepressant medications" and recommended "asking manufacturers to change the labels of 10 drugs to include stronger cautions and warnings about the need to monitor patients for the worsening of depression and the emergence of suicidal ideation, regardless of the cause of such worsening." [11] The drugs recommended for the warning are the 10 most widely used: Prozac; Zoloft; Paxil; Luvox; Celexa; Lexapro; Wellbutrin; Effexor; Serzone; and Remeron, as well as an additional 24 antidepressants.

Of the above 10 listed antidepressants under review for added warnings, only Prozac had been approved for pediatric use for the treatment of so-called major depressive disorder (MDD), and that approval for adolescent use between the ages of 7 to 17 years only was awarded by the FDA in January 2003—just one year before the hearing to determine whether these same antidepressants were responsible for the reported harmful behavior in adolescents.

But, as it is well-documented by the personal horror stories, Prozac and the other antidepressants in the SSRI class of drugs have been prescribed "off-label" (not approved by the FDA for effectiveness and safety in a particular population) to the pediatric population for more than a decade and for an ever-increasing number of psychiatric diagnoses other than the alleged mental illness of depression.

There is little doubt that each of the mental-health experts that sat on the FDA committee was well aware of the off-label prescribing long before their participation in the February 2004 hearing and, therefore, the fact that a number of families felt compelled to share the intimate and often gruesome details of young children lost to the alleged adverse effects of the antidepressants could be of little surprise. A 2003 survey by Express Scripts Inc., (the third largest pharmacy benefit manager in the United States) titled *Trends in the Use of Antidepressants in a National Sample of Commercially Insured Pediatric Patients, 1998 to 2002*, reported that the "overall prevalence of antidepressant use among children increased from 160 per 10,000 (1.6 percent) in 1998 to 240 per 10,000 (2.4 percent) in 2003," with the largest proportional increase among the youngest age group—5 years old and younger. [12] That's right. This amazing statistic is not a typographical error. Family physicians and psychiatrists are increasingly diagnosing preschool children and toddlers, whose brains still are developing, with alleged mental illnesses and prescribing extraordinarily dangerous and potentially life-threatening, mind-altering drugs that have not been approved for use in treating adolescents.

Although the February 2004 hearing had delivered a small victory to those who believe they had suffered from the adverse effects of SSRIs, at a follow-up September 2004 hearing the committee again allowed families the opportunity to share their personal stories before making a final decision on the language for the recommended label warnings.

Mark Taylor, a survivor of the deadliest school shooting at Columbine High School in Littleton, Colo., was one of many to tell the committee how SSRIs had adversely affected his life. (in part)

"I am one of the victims, one of the many victims of the SSRI antidepressant era. I took 6-13 bullets in the heart area at my high school when Eric Harris, who was, in fact, on Luvox, fired at me. They almost had to amputate my leg and my arm. My heart was missed by only one millimeter. I had three surgeries. Five years later I am still recuperating.

I had to go through all this to realize that antidepressants are dangerous for those who take them and for all of those who associate with those who take them. I hope that my testimony today shows you that you need to take action immediately before more innocent people like me and you get hurt or die horrible deaths as a result.

How are we supposed to feel safe at school, at home, on the street, at church or elsewhere if we cannot trust the FDA to do what we are paying you to do? Where were you when I got shot? You say that these antidepressants are effective. So, why did they not help Eric Harris? These drugs help increase the rage in people and cause them to do things they would not do anyway. So why didn't these so-called antidepressants not make him better? I will tell you why. It is because they don't work. We should consider antidepressants to be accomplices to the murder." [13]

Dr. Lawrence Diller, a pediatrician and author of two books: *Running on Ritalin* and *Should I Medicate My Child?* stood before the esteemed panel of his peers in support of the families he had sworn an oath to protect. (in part)

"I have prescribed psychiatric drugs to children for 26 years. I come before you as a physician in private practice with a report from the front lines, news from the primary care pediatricians and family doctors, the private practice psychiatrists and the families of the patients themselves. I am here, representing the views and the reactions of a silent majority of physicians who aren't intimately connected financially with the drug industry. All the doctors have become aware of the problems that may be developed in the early stages of SSRI treatment. They are warning the families and following children far more closely. I think it is a very good development.

However, many of the leaders in organized psychiatry and academia are publicly wringing their hands—pediatric depression is untreated they say. Now even more families will refuse medication. I find this caviling worry the height of psychiatric sanctimony. For years we were told to practice evidence-based medicine and now, when there is no evidence for SSRI effectiveness. The final blow was learning about the eight negative SSRI [antidepressant] studies in children that were never released to either the doctors or the public. This loss of credibility within the medical profession extends beyond psychiatry into all of medicine and the general public. The blame is clear: The money, power and influence of the pharmaceutical industry corrupt all. The pervasive control that the drug companies have over medical research, publications, professional organizations, doctors' practices, Congress and yes, even agencies like the FDA, is the American equivalent of a drug cartel." [14]

One month after the September 2004 hearing, and more than a decade since the self-harm issue first was raised with the FDA, the esteemed committee of mental-health experts did not go so far in protecting the public as the British, who effectively banned the use of SSRIs by adolescents, but rather issued a Public Health Advisory about the possible adverse effects of antidepressants on the adolescent population.

The FDA's conclusion was based on the "latest and best science" and "what we heard from our advisory committee last month [September 2004 hearing], as well as what many members of the public have told us." The FDA prepared to "warn the public about the increased risk of suicidal thoughts and behavior ("suicidality") in children and adolescents being treated with antidepressants." The committee "requested" pharmaceutical manufacturers to "add a 'black-box'" warning [the most serious warning placed in the labeling of a prescription medication] to the health professional labeling of all antidepressant medications to describe the risk and emphasize the need for close monitoring of patients started on these medications." [15]

The Oct. 15, 2004, FDA Public Health Advisory explained the data the committee used to come to the decision of adding black-box warnings to antidepressants:

13

*"The risk of suicidality for these drugs was identified in a combined analysis of short-term (up to four months), placebo-controlled trials of nine antidepressant drugs, including the selective serotonin reuptake inhibitors (SSRIs) and others, in children and adolescents with major depressive disorder (MDD), obsessive compulsive disorder (OCD), or other psychiatric disorders. A total of 24 trials involving over 4,400 patients were included. **The analysis showed a greater risk of suicidality during the first few months of treatment in those receiving antidepressants.** The average risk of such events on drug was 4%, twice the placebo risk of 2%."* [16]

The federal agency responsible for ensuring that drugs are safe and effective could no longer ignore the data or the public. For those experts in the psychopharmacological community who long had sung the praises of the antidepressants as psychiatric wonder drugs, it was a bitter pill to swallow. In other words, what the FDA concluded was that after a thorough review of the available clinical trial data of the top-selling antidepressants, twice as many children in pharmaceutical clinical trials taking antidepressants compared to those taking placebo (sugar pills) showed greater risk of suicidality in the first few months of treatment.

Thomas Laughren, a doctor who had participated in the 1991 hearings and now one of the reviewers and team leader for psychiatric drug products in the FDA's Division of Neuropharmacological Drug Products, admitted that of the 15 placebo-controlled clinical trials that evaluated SSRIs for treating depression in children and adolescents, only three of the trials could show positive results; the other 12 proved the mind-altering drugs were no more effective in treating the alleged mental disorder than the placebo. The results, Laughren said, "are sobering findings and certainly raise a question about the benefits of these drugs in pediatric depression." [17]

Sobering findings? Some would call it insanity that the drugs remain on the market for public consumption, especially in light of the fact that there is no science (objective, confirmable abnormality) to prove a single psychiatric mental disorder. But this point was not part of the committee's review and, worse still; the psychiatric community continues to argue that children will benefit from the psychotropic drugs—that it would be harmful if the mind-altering drugs weren't available for "treatment" in children. The question Americans have to ask is: Whose children are the acceptable risk?

Laughren's musings, though, are the very sentiments expressed by hundreds of families over a 14-year period whose loved ones did not benefit from the antidepressants but, instead, were believed by their families to have been harmed by the mind-altering drugs. Given that the majority of the clinical trials showed that the mind-altering drugs under review were no more effective than sugar pills, it would not be unfair to suggest that there is nothing "anti" about the antidepressant drugs.

The FDA found that the alleged "antidepressants" are neither safe nor effective for an unknown percentage of the adolescent population and, based on the evidence that twice as many children in clinical trials showed a greater risk of suicidality taking the antidepressants, coupled with the evidence that the antidepressants in the majority of the clinical trials were no more effective than sugar pills, the FDA had little choice but to "request" the pharmaceutical companies add the black-box warnings. The *initial* version of the warning is as follows.

Suicidality in Children and Adolescents:
"Antidepressants increase the risk of suicidal thinking and behavior (suicidality) in children and adolescents with Major Depressive Disorder (MDD) and other psychiatric disorders."

Based on the data reviewed by the committee, this seemed like appropriate language. But, when all was said and done, the FDA's final black-box warning was a skeleton of the initial language:

Suicidality in Children and Adolescents:
"Antidepressants *increased* the risk of suicidal thinking and behavior (suicidality) in *short-term studies* in children and adolescents with Major Depressive Disorder (MDD) and other psychiatric disorders." (italics mine)

Talk about shoving the knife in a little deeper! The original draft of the warning intimated that the risk was serious and ongoing within the pediatric and adolescent population. But in the final version, the FDA appears to suggest that the risk posed by the antidepressants is limited to the clinical trials or "short-term studies" that occurred in the past—as if what happens during the clinical trials doesn't carry over into the general population.

The FDA clearly took the low road on this language and the point can well be made by the simple fact that the word "increase" has been replaced to reflect the past tense in the final version and that "short-term studies" has been inserted. In what can only be described as what many believe as the standard operating procedure of putting the public's best interest behind that of the psychiatric community and pharmaceutical industry, the FDA's language changed from advising the public that "antidepressants increase the risk of suicidal thinking," to "antidepressants increased the risk of suicidal thinking and behavior in short-term studies."

This pathetic compromise looks as if the FDA is taking a bold step in advising the public that there were problems just in those darn short-term studies. If it wasn't for the explanation provided by a mouthpiece of the APA, one might rightfully conclude that the FDA committee had itself suffered from some weird collective mental deficit.

David Fassler, M.D., a child and adolescent psychiatrist and clinical associate professor of psychiatry at the University of Vermont School of Medicine and a trustee of the APA made it clear which group was responsible for the language change when, during an interview with Jim Rosack of *Clinical and Research News*, the APA spokesman said "the change in wording brings the FDA warning closer to the actual science. I'm glad they responded to the extensive and detailed input from both practicing psychiatrists and the research community. Hopefully, the FDA will consider further revisions in the future, as more long-term and follow-up data become available."

One has to wonder, though: If the APA's spokesman is right and the language is closer to the actual science, that the threat is only in the short-term clinical trials, what exactly was the reason for the FDA to warn the public about the possibility of violent behavior and self-harm? Furthermore, referring back to Graham Aldred's accounting of just the top three antidepressants, Prozac, Paxil and Zoloft, if the FDA's conclusions are accurate and the 4% greater risk of suicidality is carried over into the general public, at a minimum the number of people susceptible to the adverse reactions to the drugs could be in the millions. But, hey, the FDA's "warning" intimates that it was only those people who participated in short-term studies that experienced violent and even suicidal thoughts. Those other 68 million people taking just three of the top-selling antidepressants shouldn't have a problem. But, if the reverse logic is applied to the FDA's and APA's language, this psycho-pharma yah yah is the equivalent of saying that the percentage of the people who reportedly benefited from taking the mind-altering drug also doesn't carry over into the general population—that the benefits are limited just to the short-term studies.

Mental-health officialdom doesn't want to go down that road because the FDA's data reveal that sugar pills were as effective as the drugs in a majority of the clinical trials, but this astounding fact didn't prompt the drug approval agency to pull the mind-altering drugs from the market. This is no small point when one considers that the agency's overriding purpose is to ensure that the drugs are safe *and* effective.

The fact that the psychiatric community was behind the language change is not surprising. That Fassler would bring up "science" is quite another, important matter that lies at the heart of America's prescription psychiatric drug problem.

Nevertheless, the black-box warning, however watered down, finally ended the argument about the possible dangers of the use of SSRIs in a percentage of the adolescent population. No longer could mental-health experts dismiss the allegations surrounding the growing number of claims of adverse effects of antidepressants on an unknown percentage of the adolescent population, at the time, the only patient group reviewed by the committee. The "warning" for adults would come a few months later.

As is often the case when it comes to "fixing" federal policy, the underlying problem—the first of the two-pronged problem—whether by accident or intent, was ignored. Although necessary and most definitely a step in the right direction of providing informed consent about the risks associated with psychiatric antidepressant drugs, the action taken by the panel of mental-health experts was the equivalent of a band aid being applied to a gushing artery. While there was no doubt that the families who spoke to the FDA panel believed the mind-altering drugs prescribed to their loved ones were responsible for their deaths, unconsciously each family also clearly demonstrated that the use of an ever-increasing number of powerful, potentially life-threatening psychiatric drugs was not the originating factor that led them into their own personal abyss.

The mental-health experts charged with protecting the nation's well-being had not planned, nor were they prepared, to either debate or discuss that important factor. In the long run, anyone familiar with the growing number of suicide attempts, suicides and violence associated with psychotropic drug use could see that this small victory for American families was of little consequence without a discussion—indeed an investigation—about the legitimacy of the psychiatric diagnosis, the single factor that leads to the prescribing of the mind-altering drugs.

The pain and suffering that permeated the hearings and, on a much larger scale, the lives of countless Americans, would continue until the People could acknowledge the elephant in the room—the lack of science to support the alleged psychiatric disorders. The all important question that continually and inexplicably escapes scrutiny is: When will the psychiatric community be called upon to prove that the nearly 400 alleged psychiatric mental disorders that currently make up the DSM-IV are based in science—objective, confirmable abnormalities of the brain—and not merely *subjective* clinical diagnoses.

No diagnosis, no drugs. That is the order of events, and a close examination of the "science" that determines the nation's mental well-being is no less important than the review of the psychiatric drugs prescribed to treat the alleged psychiatric mental disorders.

[1] Anahad O'Connor, "Has the Romance Gone? Was It the Drug?" *New York Times*, May 5, 2004; Ed Silverman, "Antidepressant prescriptions show decline: Drop follows FDA meeting on links to suicides in kids, *Newark Star Ledger*, May 11, 2004; Department of Health and Human Services, Food and Drug Administration, February 2, 2004; Shankar Vedantam, "Antidepressant Use By U.S. Adults Soars," *The Washington Post*, December 3, 2004.

[2] Graham Aldred, "An Analysis of Use of Prozac, Paxil and Zoloft in USA 1988-2002," June 6, 2004.

[3] Transcript of Proceedings, Department of Health and Human Services, Public Health Service, Food and Drug Administration Psychopharmacological Drugs Advisory Committee, September 20, 1991, pp. 7-10.

[4] Ibid. pp. 13-16.

[5] Ibid. pp. 24-26.

[6] Transcript of Proceedings, Department of Health and Human Services, Public Health Service Food and Drug Administration, September 20, 1991.

[7] Transcript of Proceedings, Food and Drug Administration Center for Drug Evaluation and Research (CDER), Psychopharmacologic Drugs Advisory Committee with the Pediatric Subcommittee of the Anti-Infective Drugs Advisory Committee, February 2, 2004, pg. 1.

[8] Ibid. pp. 130-131.

[9] Ibid. pp. 87-90.

[10] Ibid. pp. 142-143.

[11] FDA Talk Paper, "FDA Issues Public Health Advisory on Cautions for Use of Antidepressants in Adults and Children." March, 22, 2004.

[12] Express Scripts, Inc., (ESI), Trends in the Use of Antidepressants in a National Sample of Commercially Insured Pediatric Patients, 1998-2002.

[13] Transcript of Proceedings, Food and Drug Administration Center for Drug Evaluation and Research (CDER), Psychopharmacologic Drugs Advisory Committee and the FDA Pediatric Advisory Committee, September 13-14, 2004, pp. 311-313.

[14] Ibid. pp. 322-325.

[15] FDA News: "FDA Launches a Multi-Pronged Strategy to Strengthen Safeguards for Children Treated With Antidepressant Medications," October 15, 2004.

[16] FDA Public Health Advisory "Suicidality in Children and Adolescents being Treated With Antidepressant Medications," October 15, 2004

[17] Thomas P. Laughren, "Background Comments for February 2, 2004 Meeting of Psychopharmacological Drugs Advisory Committee and Pediatric Subcommittee

of the Anti-Infective Drugs Advisory Committee," Food and Drug Administration Center for Drug Evaluation and Research, January 5, 2004, p 5.

Chapter Two

Psychobabble for the Masses

The ever-increasing use of dangerous, potentially life-threatening, mind-altering psychiatric drugs is a relatively new phenomenon, based solely on receiving a diagnosis of any one or number of nearly 400 alleged psychiatric mental disorders. And, because the psychiatric diagnosis must precede the prescribing of mind-altering drugs, it becomes paramount to scrutinize the very labels – the psychiatric diagnoses — that determine the mental health of the nation.

In 1961, Thomas S. Szasz, M.D., wrote the groundbreaking book *The Myth of Mental Illness: Foundations of a Theory of Personal Conduct,* exposing the fraud of modern-day psychiatry. While it has been more than 40 years since his classic work was first published, his insight remains timely. Dr. Szasz explains the difficulty the psychiatric community faces in order to gain legitimacy within the medical community. "It is important to understand clearly that modern psychiatry – and the identification of new psychiatric diseases – began not by identifying such diseases by means of the established methods of pathology, but by creating a new criterion of what constitutes disease ... thus, whereas in modern medicine new diseases were discovered, in modern psychiatry they were invented."[1]

Based on the psychiatric community's ability to convince Americans that they actually suffer from one or several of these invented diseases, a growing majority of this nation's citizens most definitely are coloring outside of the lines, and every day tens of millions of Americans are being led to believe that they need to chemically alter their brain just to function "normally."

The psychiatric community has not published a manual describing what is "normal," but, rather, the American Psychiatric Association (APA) has put pen to paper for the purpose of diagnosing what the organization considers abnormal behaviors – mental disorders – that require "treatment," which, more often than not, comes in the form of prescribing a number of dangerous, potentially life-threatening, mind-altering psychiatric drugs. And, as the theory goes, the chemicals (psychiatric drugs) will "help" the individual be "better."

The Diagnostic and Statistical Manual of Mental Disorders (DSM-IV), published by the APA, is considered the psychiatric bible of mental disorders. This most recent version, published in 1994 (a "text revision," DSM-IV-TR, was published in 2004) and weighing nearly three pounds, celebrates no less than 374 psychiatric mental disorders with accompanying criteria used by clinicians to determine an individual's mental health. On page xxi of the *DSM-IV* the definition of mental disorder is explained this way: *"...each of the mental disorders is conceptualized as a clinically significant behavioral or psychological syndrome or pattern that occurs in an individual and that is associated with present distress (e.g., a painful symptom) or disability (i.e., impairment in one or more important areas of functioning) or with a significantly increased risk of suffering death, pain, disability, or an important loss of freedom. In addition, this syndrome or pattern must not be merely an expectable and culturally sanctioned response to a particular event, for example, the death of a loved one. Whatever its original cause, it must currently be considered a manifestation of a behavioral, psychological or biological dysfunction in the individual..."*

The APA further explains in the Introduction to the *DSM-IV* that "it must be noted that DSM-IV reflects a consensus about the classification and diagnosis of mental disorders derived at the time of its initial publication." In other words, the *DSM-IV* is the result of "consensus" or agreement about the mental illness diagnosis.

The psychiatric diagnosis or mental disorder labels found in the manual are not based in science insomuch as there is no citation provided in the manual about any objective, confirmable abnormality in the brain to support a single psychiatric mental disorder. Rather, *subjective* criteria decided on by "consensus" are provided as a kind of checklist to assist the clinician in pinpointing the alleged mental disorder. For example, the criteria or checklist provided by the APA's *DSM-IV* for the alleged mental disorder Attention-Deficit Hyperactivity Disorder (ADHD) lists 18 symptoms, including the following:

1. Often fails to give close attention to details or makes careless mistakes in schoolwork, work or other activities.

2. Often has difficulty sustaining attention in tasks or play activities.

3. Often does not seem to listen when spoken to directly.

4. Often does not follow through on instructions and fails to finish schoolwork, chores or duties in the workplace.

5. Often has difficulty organizing tasks and activities.

None of the above "symptoms" of the alleged psychiatric mental disorder ADHD can be identified through medical tests such as blood work, X-rays, PET or CAT scans. In fact, the diagnosis of ADHD and any of the alleged psychiatric disorders depends completely on the clinician's observation of behavior and interpretation or opinion –including personal biases – of the information provided by the would-be patient to questions asked.

In the case of ADHD, any six of 18 symptoms must be met to be diagnosed with this alleged brain abnormality. Keeping in mind that the "mental disorder" cannot be identified by any objective, confirmable abnormality of the brain, any "normal" person, if given this information, might question the psychiatric label. This particular point seems to escape the diagnosis process, and millions of American children and an unknown number of adults, diagnosed with the alleged mental disorder, are prescribed mind-altering drugs such as the stimulant, Ritalin (active ingredient: methylphenidate), which they are assured will "help" make them "better" – more subjective jargon.

More importantly, though, one has to seriously consider just how much "better" a child, or an adult for that matter, can be after years of ingesting a prescribed psychiatric drug such as Ritalin–a stimulant (speed), and a drug the federal government, along with other world health organizations, categorizes as a Schedule II controlled substance, just like morphine, opium, cocaine and the heroin substitute methadone.

While millions of Americans have willingly accepted the diagnosis that they "suffer" from the alleged mental disorder ADHD and hundreds of other alleged mental illnesses, which they are being led to believe are real diseases of the brain, it is fair to say that most are unaware of the method in which alleged mental disorders are determined and, if they did know, would make them crazy. In fact, one doctor explained the legitimacy of psychiatric diagnosing this way: "Psychiatry is to neurology what astrology is to astronomy."

Alleged psychiatric mental disorders are not based in science, and the APA has been good enough to make this point in the Introduction to the *DSM-IV*. "...a diagnosis does not carry any necessary implications regarding the cause of the individual's mental disorder or associated impairments." For example, the *DSM-IV* explains the lack of science to support Major Depressive Episode this way: "no laboratory findings that are diagnostic of Major Depressive Episode have been identified."

This is brilliant. The deep thinkers at the APA admit there is no way of objectively diagnosing depression of any kind, let alone "major" depression, but based on subjective lists of behaviors they claim to be capable of determining an accurate level of the alleged brain abnormality: major, minimal or minor depression.

One might expect from the premier psychiatric professional organization that determines that tens of millions of Americans suffer from any number of psychiatric mental disorders at least a citation to the definitive scientific research establishing the legitimacy of the biological or neurological brain abnormality. But that is not the case. No cause(s) are provided in the manual for any of the psychiatric mental disorders, and those who "suffer" from one of the alleged mental disorders are forced to take the psychiatric organization at its word.

Wikipedia, the free internet encyclopedia, explains the *DSM* in part as "the criteria and classification system of the *DSM* are based on the majority opinion of people who represent American mental health specialists. Therefore, the content of the *DSM* does not reflect all opinions on the subject of psychopathology, nor are there any objective standards to which it can adhere. The criteria, and the way they are applied by individual clinicians are at least to some extent influenced by cultural variables. What is and what is not considered a mental disorder changes over time." [2]

One only need review the APA's reversal on homosexuality, a declassified mental disorder, to fully appreciate the speed and ease in which mental illness comes and goes in the world of psychiatry. It is important to point out that in considering the rise and fall of homosexuality in the APA's mental disorder repertoire, the reader should keep in mind that science was not part of the consideration, insomuch as there is not now nor has there ever been an objective, confirmable abnormality in the brain (or anywhere else in the body) to establish homosexuality as a bona fide disease.

Although the first manual of psychiatric mental disorders published in 1952, grouped homosexuality under personality disorders as a diagnosis of "sexual deviation," it wasn't until *DSM-II* arrived in 1968 that homosexuality was elevated and received its own diagnosis:

302 Sexual deviations. This category is for individuals whose sexual interests are directed primarily toward objects other than people of the opposite sex, toward sexual acts not usually associated with coitus, or toward coitus performed under bizarre circumstances as in necrophilia, pedophilia, sexual sadism and fetishism. Even though many find their practices distasteful, they remain unable to substitute normal sexual behavior for them. This diagnosis is not appropriate for individuals who perform deviant sexual acts because normal sexual objects are not available to them.

Homosexuality topped the list of 10 sexual deviations falling under this category. But just a few years later, when the early 1970s gay/lesbian movement took root, the APA was forced to reconsider the diagnosis, and in 1973 the board of the APA voted to remove homosexuality and replace it with "Sexual Orientation Disturbance" in the *DSM-III*. However, there was infighting among the higher-ups at the APA over this label, and in 1974 the mental disorder was again renamed and finally included in the *DSM-III* as Ego-dystonic Homosexuality (EDH). By 1987 EDH was eliminated from the updated *DSM-III-R* (the revised third edition). Today, the most recent psychiatric manual of alleged mental disorders, the *DSM-IV*, does not directly mention homosexuality, but rather provides a category "Gender Identity Disorder" with a subcategory Sexual Disorder Not Otherwise Specified (302.9; page 538), for those individuals who experience "persistent and marked distress about sexual orientation."

The above revisions to, and ultimate elimination from, the *DSM* were not carried out by committees considering medical or scientific data regarding any known biological or neurological cause of an alleged mental illness because, like every other alleged psychiatric mental disorder, there is no objective, confirmable abnormality in the brain that identifies homosexuality. Rather, the APA's reversal was in response to increased public pressure applied by a growing and very vocal segment of the population that most certainly did not accept that their sexual orientation was due to an abnormality of the brain. With no science to back up the psychiatric claims, the APA had little choice but to acquiesce or face a public showdown which would have forced the powerful organization to prove an objective, confirmable abnormality for the alleged mental illness, possibly opening the door to scientific, research-based study of the other alleged mental illnesses.

Given the results of the skirmish over labeling gay men and lesbians as mentally ill, one can only imagine what would happen if the APA was forced to prove to the tens of millions of Americans diagnosed with ADHD or one of the other nearly four hundred psychiatric mental disorders that they actually suffer from a neurologic or biologic abnormality of the brain.

But for the psychiatric community, confirmation of objective, confirmable abnormalities in the brain has never been a scientific standard to be met when considering what constitutes mental illness. The records from St. Elizabeth's Hospital in Washington, D.C., once the nation's premier psychiatric facility are, perhaps, a good barometer to show that psychiatric diagnosing has progressed little if at all in the last 150 years. It is reported that, at a minimum, 125,000 patients were admitted to the psychiatric hospital and a review of the admitting books describes the illness, symptoms and cause of the mental disease:

Patient #2385 – disease: chronic dementia; cause: masturbation.
Patient #2395 – disease: acute mania; cause: masturbation.
Patient #7827 – disease: chronic melancholia; cause: intemperance.
Patient #7838 – disease: acute melancholia; cause: intemperance.
Patient #6896 – disease: acute melancholia; cause: poverty.
Patient #6889 – disease: acute mania; cause: prison life.

Is it possible that masturbation, intemperance, poverty and prison life cause mental instability? Sure. Are any of these "causes" brain diseases? No. And, although there were no individual case files available for review, it is difficult to know what the then-experts in psychiatry believed was excessive masturbation, the level of poverty or the duration of prison life that led to and qualified patients as having the alleged mental "disease." The same questions can be asked about today's psychiatric diagnosing.

One only has to leisurely peruse the hundreds of alleged psychiatric mental illnesses catalogued in the *DSM-IV* to see that in the last 150 years the names of alleged psychiatric mental illnesses may have changed and even greatly increased in number but, despite major advances in medicine and science, the causes of alleged psychiatric mental disorders remain elusive.

For example, the APA on page 50 of the *DSM-IV* lists *"Mathematics Disorder (315.1)"* in part as "mathematical ability that falls substantially below that expected for the individual's chronological age, measured intelligence, and age-appropriate education." And, for those individuals who don't have problems with numbers but can't seem to put their thoughts on paper, the APA included on page 51 of the *DSM-IV* the mental disorder, *"Disorder of Written Expression (315.2)."* A child can be labeled with this mental illness, as in the case of Mathematics Disorder, "if writing skills fall substantially below those expected given the individual's chronological age, measured intelligence, and age-appropriate education."

In both of the above cases of "mental disorders" the APA advises that they usually are apparent by the second or third grade. There is no discussion about the scientific cause(s) of these alleged mental illnesses, such as precisely where in the brain the objective, confirmable abnormality that is "mathematics disorder" or "written expression disorder" can be found. Is it possible that some kids "get" math and some don't? That some kids are just better writers than others? That tutoring may be the answer? No, apparently not and yet the intellectual giants of mental health present not even a shred of scientific evidence to support a neurologic or biologic abnormality of the brain for either of these alleged mental disorders.

Listed under the "Attention-Deficit and Disruptive Behavior Disorders" is "Conduct Disorder" (312.8), on page 85 of the DSM-IV. "Conduct Disorder" is "a repetitive and persistent pattern of behavior in which basic rights of others or major age-appropriate social norms or rules are violated." And, not to be confused with "Conduct Disorder," there is "Oppositional Defiant Disorder" (313.81) on page 91 of the *DSM-IV,* which features a "recurrent pattern of negativistic, defiant, disobedient and hostile behavior toward authority figures that persists for at least six months." This category is so subjectively broad that anyone who dared to question the psychiatric label – anyone who verbalized the nonsense of it, could be diagnosed with the alleged mental illness.

But in reviewing the above mental disorders, one has to wonder whether "conduct disorder" isn't negative, defiant, disobedient and hostile behavior? And if it is all of these things, wouldn't it make it difficult for any clinician to accurately diagnose between the two alleged mental disorders? This is where science would come in handy. Diagnosing either of these "mental disorders" is based on a subjective understanding of the information provided to the clinician, not whether there is an objective, confirmable abnormality of the brain.

Moving along to some of the "Substance-Related Disorders" there is that well-known mental illness, "Caffeine Intoxication" (305.90) on page 212 of the *DSM-IV.* "Caffeine Intoxication" occurs with the "recent consumption of caffeine and five or more symptoms that develop during, or shortly after, caffeine use. Symptoms that can appear following the ingestion of as little as 100 mg of caffeine per day include restlessness, nervousness, excitement, insomnia, flushed face, diuresis, and gastrointestinal complaints." However, according to the *DSM-IV*, regardless of whether one actually ingests these levels of caffeine, "intoxication may *not* occur despite high caffeine intake because of the development of tolerance." (italics mine)

Apparently, what we're being told here is that if no symptoms are being displayed then the mental disorder doesn't exist. Or, the patient *is* suffering from this mental disorder but doesn't know it because there are no visible symptoms. But in the event that one is "intoxicated" from overabundant caffeine use and decides the best course of action is to stop ingesting products which contain caffeine, the *DSM-IV* also has graciously provided an explanation for the alleged mental illness "Caffeine Withdrawal." This particular mental illness is listed on page 708 of the psychiatric manual under "Criteria Sets and Axes Provided for Further Study." Apparently, "the essential feature (of caffeine withdrawal) is a characteristic withdrawal syndrome due to the abrupt cessation of, or reduction in, the use of caffeine-containing products after prolonged daily use."

It's a logical assumption that anyone who daily drinks large quantities of coffee and then abruptly ceases might experience withdrawal, but is it a psychiatric mental disorder in need of psychiatric treatment and/or drugs? Moreover, one has to wonder just how many Americans stopped drinking coffee and then ran in a panic to their psychiatrists seeking help from the suffering of caffeine intoxication/withdrawal, which apparently led to the alleged mental disorders being included in the manual. The truth is, like all of the above alleged psychiatric mental disorders, "caffeine intoxication" and "caffeine withdrawal" are not based in science - objective, confirmable abnormalities of the brain.

One of the problems with taking the *DSM-IV* seriously (apart from the fact that it isn't based in science) is that the manual covers the psychiatric bases so completely that depending on one's alleged mental affliction, you're damned if you do and damned if you don't. Let me explain. Listed under Substance-Related Disorders are subcategories such as Alcohol Intoxication (303.00) page 196, Amphetamine Intoxication (292.89) page 207, Cannabis Intoxication (292.89) page 217, Cocaine Intoxication (292.89) page 223 and Inhalant Intoxication (292.89) page 239 to name just a few.

Each of these alleged mental disorders comes with clinical criteria to assist in the appropriate diagnosis, which apparently allows for the clinician to recommend appropriate treatment.

Here's the rub: Once a patient is diagnosed with one or several of these substance-related psychiatric mental disorders and decides to kick the habit, more often than not the patient will experience symptoms of withdrawal, which the APA also considers a mental disorder (Alcohol Withdrawal (291.8) page 197, Amphetamine Withdrawal (292.0) page 208, Cocaine Withdrawal (292.0) page 225). Apparently, there are no withdrawal symptoms associated with cannabis and inhalants as the APA has not included withdrawal from these substances in the manual of mental disorders.

The bottom line appears to be, at least according to the deep thinkers at the APA, if you use, abuse or experience withdrawal from one of the above substances, with the exception of pot or glue, you are suffering from a mental illness. What gets lost in the APA's psychobabble is not whether these substances chemically alter the mind. Illegal substances, as well as the now socially acceptable prescription psychiatric mind-altering drugs the nation swallows everyday, alter the chemicals in the brain. What is in question is the APA's ability to provide scientific data to support that the use, abuse and withdrawal of these substances is due to an objective, confirmable abnormality of the brain.

One of my personal favorites is the mental disorder "Nicotine Dependence" (305.10) explained in part on page 243 of the manual as "...many individuals who use nicotine take nicotine to relieve or to avoid withdrawal symptoms when they wake up in the morning or after being in a situation where use is restricted (e.g., at work or on an airplane). Individuals who smoke and other individuals who use nicotine are likely to find that they use up their supply of cigarettes or other nicotine-containing products faster than originally intended." Wow, now there's some serious science!

As with the other substance-related psychiatric disorders, if the user/abuser curtails the use of nicotine, they then may be diagnosed with the alleged mental disorder "Nicotine Withdrawal" (292.0) page 244. That's right, you guessed it, withdrawal occurs "after the abrupt cessation of, or reduction in, the use of nicotine-containing products following a prolonged period (at least several weeks) of daily use." This appears to be a no-brainer (no pun intended) and the same could be said about withdrawal from sugar and a host of other products. But even here the APA covers its bases so completely that they've added the catch-all category "Other (or Unknown) Substance-Related Disorders" with the subcategory, "Other (or Unknown) Substance Withdrawal" (304.80) pages 270-271.

At this point the reader may have noticed that the focus has been on little-known alleged mental disorders; no mention has been made of the more common psychiatric diagnosis' such as "depression" "schizophrenia," "obsessive-compulsive disorder" or "bi-polar disorder" – the alleged mental illnesses from which tens of millions of Americans are reported to "suffer." The reason is simple. Like the above-mentioned alleged mental disorders, there is no known objective, confirmable abnormality of the brain for depression, schizophrenia, obsessive-compulsive disorder or bi-polar disorder. These mental disorders, like all the other alleged psychiatric mental disorders, are determined by the "experts" in mental health based on agreement of subjective criteria – lists of behavioral symptoms that essentially are opinions.

In fact, there are a growing number of experts in mental health that refuse to accept the *DSM-IV* as a legitimate tool of scientific diagnosis, including Margaret Hagen, author of *Whores of the Court*, who dismisses the *DSM* saying "given their farcical 'empirical' procedures for arriving at new disorders with their associated symptoms list, where does the American Psychiatric Association get off claiming a scientific, research-based foundation for its diagnostic manual? This is nothing more than science by decree. They say it is science, so it is." [3]

Jeffrey A. Schaler, Ph.D., explains the legitimacy of the *DSM* this way: "the notion of scientific validity, though not an act, is related to fraud. Validity refers to the extent to which something represents or measures what it purports to represent or measure. When diagnostic measures do not represent what they purport to represent, we say that the measure lacks validity. If a business transaction or trade rested on such a lack of validity, we might say that the lack of validity was instrumental in a commitment of fraud. The *Diagnostic and Statistical*

Manual (DSM-IV) published by the American Psychiatric Association and used by licensed psychotherapists throughout the country is notorious for low scientific validity. Yet it is instrumental in securing insurance reimbursement for psychotherapy services..." [4]

And Herb Kutchins of California State University, Sacramento, and Stuart A. Kirk of the University of California, Los Angeles, authors of *Making Us Crazy: The Psychiatric Bible and the Creation of Mental Disorders*, tell us that "the developers of *DSM* assume that if a group of psychiatrists agree on a list of atypical [new] behaviors, the behaviors constitute a valid mental disorder. Using this approach, creating mental disorders can become a parlor game in which clusters of all kinds of behaviors (i.e. syndromes) can be added to the manual." [5]

Lynne Rosewater, a psychologist who attended one session where new disorders were being considered and which was being presided over by one of the *DSM's* leading architects, psychiatrist Robert Spitzer, recalls that "they were having a discussion for a criterion about Masochistic Personality Disorder and Bob Spitzer's wife says, 'I do that sometimes,' and he says, 'Okay, take it out.'"

"You watch this," says Rosewater, "and say, 'Wait a second, we don't have a right to criticize them because this is a science?'"[6]

Former Assistant District Attorney in California Lawrence Stevens says, "If mental illness were really an illness in the same sense that physical illnesses are illnesses, the idea of deleting homosexuality or anything else from the categories of illness by having a vote would be as absurd as a group of physicians voting to delete cancer or measles from the concept of disease." [7]

Dr. Sydney Walker III, author of *A Dose of Sanity*, wrote "the American Psychiatric Association is literally built on a foundation of drug money," which that influence, he says, "has focused on expanding the number of 'psychiatric disorders' recognized by the APA, and the number of drug treatments recommended for these disorders. After all, every *DSM* 'diagnosis,' is a potential gold mine for pharmaceutical firms." [8]

Dr. Thomas Dorman, a member of the Royal College of Physicians of the United Kingdom and fellow of the Royal College of Physicians in Canada, says, "In short, the whole business of creating psychiatric categories of 'disease,' formalizing them with consensus, and subsequently ascribing diagnostic codes to them, which in turn leads to their use for insurance billing, is nothing but an extended racket furnishing psychiatry a pseudo-scientific aura. The perpetrators are, of course, feeding at the public trough." [9]

Paula Caplan, Ph.D., Professor of Applied Psychology at the Ontario Institute for Studies in Education and author of several books including *They Say You're Crazy: How the World's Most Powerful Psychiatrists Decide Who's Normal,* explains: "I served on two of the committees that were charged with writing the current edition [of the *DSM-IV*] and I resigned from both of those committees because, as a clinical and research psychologist who among other things specializes in research methodology and psychiatric assessment, I was horrified when I saw what is done with the science by the members of the *DSM* groups. At various times I firsthand saw them ignore the scientific research, distort good scientific research and can even say I saw them lie about good scientific research. I also saw them produce or use research that was poorly done when the results were said to come from that poor research suited their purposes. So when they say that it is scientifically based it couldn't be further from the truth."

And finally, Dr. Robert Spitzer, the well-known architect of the DSM admitted in the Jan. 3, 2005, edition of the *New Yorker* magazine, "To say that we've solved the reliability problems is just not true. It's [*DSM*] been improved. But if you're in a situation with a general clinician it's certainly not very good."[10] Given that the majority of prescriptions for mind-altering antidepressants now are written by general practitioners – the family physician – Spitzer's admission is a frightening commentary on the accuracy of psychiatric diagnosing.

Some physicians, so disturbed by the deterioration of their profession, have felt compelled to put pen to paper regarding their observations of the APA, one going so far as to resign from membership with the professional organization. The following excerpts are representative of what a growing number of doctors believe to be pervasive throughout the APA.

The late Loren Mosher, M.D., resigned his membership from the APA in a letter addressed to Rodrigo Munzo, (former) president of the APA, in December 1998 saying in part:

After nearly three decades as a member it is with a mixture of pleasure and disappointment that I submit this letter of resignation from the American Psychiatric Association. The major reason for this action is my belief that I am actually resigning from the American Psychopharmacological Association; the organization's true identity requires no change in the acronym.

Unfortunately, APA reflects, and reinforces, in word and deed, our drug dependent society. Yet, it helps wage war on drugs (sic). Dual Diagnosis clients are a major problem for the field but not because of the good drugs we prescribe. Bad ones are those that are obtained mostly without prescription. APA likes only those drugs from which it can derive a profit – directly or indirectly. This is not a group for me. In my view, psychiatry has been almost completely bought out by the drug companies. The APA could not continue without the pharmaceutical company support of meetings, symposia, workshops, journal advertising, grand rounds luncheons, unrestricted educational grants, etc.

Finally, why must the APA pretend to know more than it does? DSM-IV is the fabrication upon which psychiatry seeks acceptance by medicine in general. Insiders know it is more a political than scientific document. The issue is what do the categories tell us? Do they in fact accurately represent the person with a problem? They don't, and can't, because there are no external validating criteria for psychiatric diagnoses. There is neither a blood test nor specific anatomic lesions for any major psychiatric disorder. So, where are we? APA as an organization has implicitly (sometimes explicitly as well) bought into a theoretical hoax.

Alex Braiman, M.D., after receiving a 50-year distinguished fellow award from the APA in 2004, wrote a letter to the editor of *Psychiatric News*. Dr. Braiman's thoughts, under the title "One-Trick Training," were published in the Aug. 6, 2004, edition of the professional psychiatric journal (in part):

"After receiving my 50-year distinguished fellow award at APA's 2004 annual meeting in May, there was time for thought on the flight

back to New Mexico and my practice. APA has become a polarized organization, perhaps a reflection of the larger society, but it has tilted too far toward the advocacy of unsupported "biologic" diagnostic and treatment practices that corrode its efficacy and leadership.

It is ironic that we are witnessing serious challenges to the scientific integrity of studies supporting the FDA approval of the SSRI class of antidepressants at a time when an unsilent majority of us go along with the pretense that this is evidence-based psychiatry.

It is too easy to fault drug companies. There are too many of us whose integrity has been compromised by grant support or honoraria for the rest of us to be able to trust their advice. I consider myself fortunate to be able to continue to practice psychiatry now that I am retired from teaching and lucky that I received my award before the name APA changes, perhaps to the American Bipolar Association."

The level of frustration, disappointment and disillusionment expressed by the above doctors about the APA and its diagnostic criteria represents a level of honesty and integrity that an increasing number of professionals in the field are concluding is an accurate portrayal of the organization that determines the nation's mental health. The vast majority of mental-health professionals, and the public, private and government-run organizations and institutions they represent, through what could be construed as misleading and deceptive advertising and information campaigns continue, despite no scientific proof of a neurological or biological abnormality for any of the psychiatric diagnoses', to push the neurologic-biologic line.

For example, the federal government's National Institute of Mental Health (NIMH), operates an extensive website, allowing access to an abundance of information about any number of the alleged mental illnesses, including "depression" and "schizophrenia." Under the category "depression" NIMH offers four pages of information titled **"The Invisible Disease: Depression"** which explains that "Depression is a serious medical condition. In contrast to the normal emotional experiences of sadness, loss, or passing mood states, clinical depression is persistent and can interfere significantly with an individual's ability to function..."

NIMH further explains the treatment options for depression including antidepressant medications, certain types of psychotherapy, cognitive-behavioral therapy and even electroconvulsive (electroshock) therapy. Then, listed under "Research Findings" NIMH, rather than provide the objective, confirmable abnormality in the brain that apparently causes the *"invisible disease,"* offers citations to research about a number of *possibilities* for the cause of depression, including neural circuits, genetics, stressful life events and the hypothalamic-pituitary-adrenal axis. In other words, despite no known cause for depression, the deep thinkers at NIMH persist in misleading the public about the cause of depression by calling it the *"invisible disease."*

The same tactic is used by NIMH in describing "Schizophrenia" when the institute explains it is ***"a chronic, severe, and disabling brain disease."*** But even in its own literature, NIMH blows the "brain-disease" theory when it reports on its website: "Research is gradually leading to new and safer medications and unraveling the complex causes of the disease." The nation's best and brightest at NIMH are still "unraveling the complex causes?" Moreover, NIMH further adds on its website: "there is no known single cause of schizophrenia. Many diseases, such as heart disease, result from an interplay of genetic, environmental, and behavioral factors; this may be the case for schizophrenia as well. Scientists do not yet understand all of the factors necessary to produce schizophrenia, but all the tools of modern biomedical research are being used to search for genes, critical moments in brain development, and environmental factors that may lead to the illness."

Virtually two pages into NIMH's explanation of Schizophrenia, the authors stop using "brain disease" and begin referring to Schizophrenia as an "illness." More importantly, despite the fact that NIMH first explains Schizophrenia as a "chronic, severe, and disabling brain disease," the federal agency has no evidence to support the objective, confirmable abnormality in the brain which would validate the disease, and NIMH openly admits that it does not know and, in fact, still is "unraveling the causes." But, like the APA, not having any scientific evidence to support the psychiatric brain disease, doesn't stop the agency from calling the behavior a "disease." That people are suffering isn't in question; that they suffer from an objective, confirmable brain "disease" is.

But while one federal government agency plays fast and loose with what constitutes "disease," the federal Center for Disease Control and Prevention (CDC), offers no confirmation of the "brain disease" for any childhood psychiatric diagnoses. For example, the CDC website offers categories for review, including "Childhood Diseases." One need only peruse the list of childhood diseases listed by the CDC to notice that not a single psychiatric diagnosis is listed.

If, in fact, the APA and NIMH are correct and the psychiatric diagnoses are real diseases of the brain, wouldn't one expect the United States' leading watchdog of disease to at least list the psychiatric diseases? It appears that the CDC requires a higher standard of what constitutes disease than does the APA and NIMH. The FDA, on the other hand, apparently cannot decide what to call mental illness. In an Oct. 27, 2003, "Talk Paper" the FDA refers to Major Depressive Disorder (MDD) as a "serious condition," but in a March 22, 2004, FDA Public Health Advisory, the agency that approves the use of mind-altering drugs to treat alleged mental illnesses describes depression as "the underlying disease." It appears that at the FDA the confusion in describing the alleged mental disorder of depression depends on the individual writing the press release.

But the fraud of psychiatric brain disease doesn't end with governmental agencies and private professional organizations; the pharmaceutical companies also have jumped on to the "brain disease" bandwagon. For instance, Eli Lilly and Co., the makers of Prozac, the first Selective Serotonin Reuptake Inhibitor (SSRI), list **"Disease Information"** at the top of its website for information about depression, one of the illnesses the mind-altering drug allegedly "treats." And like the APA and NIMH, Lilly also cannot support depression being a brain disease but, rather, reports that it may be due to "severe psychological stress, a physical illness or condition, medications and alcohol or drug abuse." Lilly also adds that "sometimes depression appears to have no trigger." But Lilly's crescendo is the well-known but unproven "chemical imbalance" theory. The makers of Prozac state: "While depression is not fully understood, a growing amount of evidence supports the view that people with depression *may* have an imbalance of the brain's neurotransmitters…" (italics mine)

This is the crux of the problem of subjective psychiatric diagnosing. "While depression is not fully understood," and, therefore, it cannot be known if the psychiatric diagnosis is an abnormality (disease) of the brain, the APA, NIMH and the makers of the dangerous psychiatric mind-altering drugs that reportedly "treat" the alleged mental illnesses have no problem referring to the alleged mental disorders as a "disease." And, after years of convincing the public that tens of millions are afflicted with one of the alleged psychiatric mental disorders, the most recent explanation physicians, researchers and scientists can come up with in its never-ending search for scientific legitimacy of psychiatric diagnosing is the alleged phantom "chemical imbalance."

[1] Thomas S. Szasz, M.D., The Myth of Mental Illness: Foundations of a Theory of Personal Conduct, (Harper & Row, Publishers), P.12.

[2] http://en.wikipedia.org/wiki/DSM

[3] Margaret Hagen, Ph.D., Whores of the Court, The Fraud of Psychiatric Testimony and the Rape of American Justice, (Harper Collins Publishers, Inc., New York, 1997), p. 42.

[4] Jeffrey A. Schaler, Ph.D., Good Therapy, *Mental Health Net – The InterPsych Newsletter*, Volume 2, Issue 7, Aug-Sep, 1995, Internet URL: http://mentalhelp.net/ipn/ipn27d.htm.

[5] Herb Kutchins & Stuart A. Kirk, Making Us Crazy: The Psychiatric Bible and the Creation of Mental Disorders, (The Free Press, New York, 1997), p. 252.

[6] Susan Fauldi, Backlash: The Undeclared War Against Women, (New York: Crown, 1991), p.361.

[7] Lawrence Stevens, J.D., Does Mental Illness Exist? undated article.

[8] Sydney Walker III, M.D., A Dose of Sanity, (John Wiley & Sons, Inc., New York, 1996), p.228.

[9] Thomas A. Dorman, M.D., Toxic Psychiatry, The Role of Psychiatry in Mind Control, http://www.dormanpub.com.

[10] Alix Spiegel, The Dictionary of Disorder, How One Man Revolutionized Psychiatry, *The New Yorker*, January 3, 2005

Chapter Three

Chemical Imbalance:
A Measure of Madness?

It's hard to argue with the numbers, however underreported they may be. America, the nation of tough, indefatigable people that tamed the West and were first to land a man on the moon, has become an ever-increasing population of mentally ill patients. In fact, one recent Harvard University study predicts that one-half of all Americans—150 million people—will have a mental illness sometime in their life. [1]

The scattered data tell us that, at minimum, tens of millions of Americans currently "suffer" from one or several alleged mental illnesses; we know this to be so because mental-health experts have told us we are mentally ill. But how do the experts deduce the extent of the nation's mental health? Well, they just ask us.

As is clearly demonstrated by the APA's *DSM-IV*, mental illness is *not* determined by medical laboratory tests, such as blood work, X-rays, CAT or PET scans, or even MRIs. Rather, the nation's mental health is determined by answers given in response to a set of questions matched against predetermined subjective psychiatric disorder criteria—lists of behavioral symptoms.

Despite there being no known objective biological or neurological test to determine any alleged psychiatric mental illness, Americans are being led to believe that psychiatric disorders are actual "diseases" of the brain, with the most obvious misconception being the mistaken belief that mental disorders are derived from a "chemical imbalance" in the brain.

But what defines a "chemical imbalance?" As the theory goes, low levels of serotonin (or a number of other naturally occurring chemicals) in the brain cause symptoms of depression or a number of other alleged psychiatric disorders. Serotonin is a neurotransmitter, a naturally occurring chemical that nerve cells use to communicate with each other. If serotonin is at a low level in the brain, then the cells that need it to function don't respond very well and the alleged psychiatric disorder occurs. If the serotonin is increased, the cells can function properly and the "imbalance" is corrected. Voila! The chemical imbalance theory.

Here's the problem with the theory: To date, there is no test available to determine a chemical balance in the brain and, therefore, making it impossible to determine whether the naturally occurring chemicals in the brain are out of balance. Nevertheless, despite there being not a single objective biological or neurological test to determine whether the chemicals in the brain are in or out of balance, the theory continues and people are led to believe they "suffer" from some alleged mental illness because of this "chemical imbalance." And the pharmaceutical companies that manufacture the mind-altering drugs to "correct" the imbalance continue to push the theory.

For example, Pfizer—the pharmaceutical company that manufactures Zoloft, one of the SSRI antidepressants listed by the FDA for "black box" warnings—until July 2005 reported on the company's Zoloft website: "Although the way Zoloft works for depression, panic disorder, Obsessive Compulsive Disorder (OCD), and Post Traumatic Stress Disorder (PTSD) is not completely understood, what is understood is that **Zoloft is a medicine that helps correct the chemical imbalance of serotonin in the brain...**" [2] (emphasis mine)

Any one reading the company's website might be persuaded to believe that the pharmaceutical company knows what it is talking about, that there is some basis in fact to support such a definitive statement. After all, the company was not qualifying the statement with language such as "might," "may" or "believes" Zoloft helps correct the chemical imbalance. No, Pfizer was stating unequivocally that its mind-altering drug "helps correct the chemical imbalance of serotonin in the brain." And the company is selling a mind-altering drug that is intended to "treat" one of the stated psychiatric diagnoses, so one might believe, and even expect, the pharmaceutical company to have some objective, confirmable evidence that a "chemical imbalance" exists. While it is clear that Pfizer believes a "chemical imbalance" exists in the brain (why else would the company make the statement that its drug helps correct the imbalance), there is no definitive objective biological or neurological evidence to support this claim and numerous respected doctors and researchers have just as definitively made this clear. The following are just a sample of such statements.

"Although a physician may tell a patient that a chemical imbalance causes their depression, the physician would be hard-pressed to provide any evidence to support this claim. There is no test available that would demonstrate that any patient has a biological depression as opposed to any other type, or even that such biological depressions exist." Antonuccio et al., *Psychiatric Times*, 12:8 August 2000.

"There are no external validating criteria for psychiatric diagnoses. There is neither blood test nor specific anatomic lesions for any major psychiatric disorder."

Loren Mosher, M.D., former chief of the NIMH Center for the Study of Schizophrenia.

"Despite more than two hundred years of intensive research, no commonly diagnosed psychiatric disorders have been proven to be either genetic or biological in origin, including schizophrenia, major depression, manic-depressive disorder, the various anxiety disorders, and childhood disorders such as attention-deficit hyperactivity. At present there are no known biochemical imbalances in the brain of typical psychiatric patients—until they are given psychiatric drugs."

Peter Breggin, M.D., *Brain Disabling Treatments in Psychiatry* (Springer Publishing Co., New York, 1997), p.5.

"Throughout "mental health" psychiatrists and other physicians as well, use the term "chemical imbalance" to mean "disorder" / "disease" / "sickness" / "illness" when there is never an abnormality on any kind of examination or test. Such is the total 100% fraud of psychiatry's "chemical imbalances"— psychiatry's way of making patients of normals."

Fred Baughman, M.D., Neurologist; Fellow, American Academy of Neurology, July 8, 2005.

"There is still no valid biological test for depression." Connie S. Chan, Ph.D., *If It Runs in Your Family: Depression*, 1993 Bantam Books, p.106.

"There are no tests available for assessing the chemical status of a living person's brain." Elliot S. Valenstein, Ph.D., *Blaming the Brain* (The Free Press, New York, 1998), p. 4.

"...Modern psychiatry has yet to convincingly prove the genetic/biologic cause of any single mental illness. Patients have been diagnosed with 'chemical imbalances' despite the fact that no test exists to support such a claim, and ... there is no real conception of what a correct chemical balance would look like." David Kaiser, M.D., "Commentary: Against Biologic Psychiatry," *Psychiatric Times*, Dec. 1996.

"There is no blood or other biological test to ascertain the presence or absence of a mental illness, as there is for most bodily diseases. If such a test were developed (for what, theretofore, had been considered a psychiatric illness), then the condition would cease to be a mental illness and would be classified, instead, as a symptom of a bodily disease." Dr. Thomas Szasz, professor of psychiatry emeritus, 2002.

"Remember that no biochemical, neurological, or genetic markers have been found for attention deficit disorder, oppositional defiant disorder, depression, schizophrenia, anxiety, compulsive alcohol and drug abuse, overeating, gambling, or any other so-called mental illness, disease or disorder." Bruce D. Levine, Ph.D., *Common Sense Rebellion: Debunking Psychiatry, Confronting Society* (Continuum, New York, 2001) p. 277.

And, perhaps, the most conspicuous and explosive admission that there is no way to test for a "chemical imbalance" in the brain came from the grand pooh-bah of psychiatry, Dr. Steven Sharfstein, president of the American Psychiatric Association, APA, when, in an interview in *People* magazine (July 11, 2005) the top shrink admitted **"we do not have a clean-cut lab test"** (to determine a chemical imbalance in the brain). Truth be told, Sharfstein is fully aware that there is *no* test available, let alone "a clean-cut" test, to determine chemical levels in a living brain, but in what can only be described as a continuance of the fraud perpetrated by the APA about the "chemical imbalance" theory, the nation's top shrink provides a clever response, leaving one to believe that there is *some* objective lab test, just not a "clean-cut" test.

Nevertheless, getting back to Pfizer, given that the above respected doctors and researchers, including the APA, state that not only is there no way to "test" for a chemical imbalance but also that there is no objective, confirmable, evidence to support that chemical imbalance is a proven abnormality of the brain, why would Pfizer state that its drug helps correct the alleged imbalance? Well, before getting into Pfizer's and other pharmaceutical companies' comments on "chemical imbalance," there are several interesting items of note on Pfizer's website as of July 2005, the first of which is that the company was stating up front and quite clearly that it is not sure how Zoloft works in the treatment of the alleged mental disorders for which the drug has been approved: "Although the way Zoloft works for depression, panic disorder, OCD and PTSD is not completely understood..."

While one can appreciate the company's honesty in admitting that it is unsure exactly how its drug works in the brain for the treatment of the listed alleged mental disorders, Pfizer does not go so far as to provide the public with the level of its understanding of the way Zoloft works for the alleged mental disorders. The confusing, and perhaps misleading, word used by the pharmaceutical company is "completely," leaving one to believe there is *some* level of objective understanding. Could it be the company is 60 percent sure and 40 percent unsure, or is it 20 percent sure and 80 percent unsure? Given that Pfizer has failed to reveal to the public its precise level of understanding, it seems possible, and even probable given that there is no known cause for any of the alleged psychiatric mental illnesses the drug is reported to "treat," that the level of understanding about how Zoloft works in the brain for the treatment of the stated alleged mental illnesses is zero.

Since there is no objective, confirmable method or test for determining any of the nearly 400 alleged mental disorders, making it extraordinarily difficult (if not impossible) to effectively treat the unknown, at least Pfizer is being honest about the drug the company is hawking. The company doesn't know how its drug works in the treatment of depression because no company, no doctor, no association of mental health experts has a definitive answer for the cause of depression. This kind of honesty has to make one wonder how many people diagnosed with an alleged mental illness would take the mind-altering drug had their physicians told them "Hey, you know the pharmaceutical company that sells this drug doesn't completely understand how this drug works in your brain, but they say it does and you'll feel 'better.'" But this information is not regularly divulged by the family physician prescribing the mind-altering drug.

More importantly, though, since the pharmaceutical company was publicly stating that its mind-altering drug "helps correct the chemical imbalance of serotonin in the brain," then it seems logical, and the public would trust, that the company is aware of some demonstrable objective biological/neurological test that proves there is a chemical imbalance in the brain. And because of the precise wording of Pfizer's statement, the company was further implying that patients diagnosed with one of the stated psychiatric disorders that Zoloft "treats" have apparently not only tested positive for this chemical imbalance, but also that a demonstrable percentage of the chemical deficiency can be measured and cited, or why would an individual need the "treatment"—an increase of the brain chemicals—that reportedly are out of balance?

In other words, if such a "chemical imbalance" test did exist one might think of it like a person being in an automobile accident, having lost a significant amount of blood and in need of a certain number of replacement pints of blood. In the case of the "chemical imbalance," one might require so many micrograms/milligrams or such of serotonin to correct the brain chemicals reportedly out of balance. But such a test does not exist, and we know this to be true because the FDA has never approved for sale a "test" that measures chemical levels in the brain.

Even on a more basic level, would it not seem logical that if such a test existed that the pharmaceutical companies that manufacture the drugs to "correct" the "imbalance" would also sell the test that determines not only that there is a "chemical imbalance" but also the level or degree of imbalance? Clearly there would be millions if not billions of dollars to be made on such a test, but no such test is mentioned by Pfizer or on any of the websites for the antidepressant drugs sold to "treat" the alleged mental disorders allegedly caused by a "chemical imbalance."

There always are people who want to believe in the "chemical imbalance" theory, regardless of the evidence or, in this case, the lack of evidence. In fact, the APA, governmental bodies, pharmaceutical companies and private mental health organizations have spent billions on advertising campaigns to educate and reassure those afflicted with the reported psychiatric mental illnesses that it isn't their fault and that they shouldn't be stigmatized.

So for those skeptics that still believe that the "chemical imbalance" is more than a theory—indeed a hypothesis—there is one sure-fire way to know the truth on a very personal level: Ask your treating physician or psychiatrist for a paper copy of the results of the test that was conducted to measure your brain chemical levels. Something along the lines of: grossly, minimally, or just a smidge out of balance, providing the physician a template to determine the necessary dosage and, more importantly, the duration of treatment. And, one might assume, this test presumably would also be used at the completion of treatment to determine if the chemical "imbalance" had been sufficiently corrected or balanced.

Researchers would be unable to locate a single psychiatric drug user capable of providing such results. It is fair to say that if objective, confirmable proof of a neurological "chemical imbalance" were required prior to filling a prescription for any of the psychiatric mind-altering antidepressants that reportedly "correct" the "chemical imbalance" in the brain, not a single prescription would be written because to date the only known method of determining chemical levels in the brain is during autopsy.

Jonathan Leo, associate professor of anatomy at Western University of Health Sciences and author of *Broken Brains or Flawed Studies? A Critical Review of ADHD Neuroimaging Research*, hit the nail on the head about the legitimacy of "chemical imbalance" when he explained in his 2004 paper "The Biology of Mental Illness": *"If a psychiatrist says you have a shortage of a chemical, ask for a blood test and watch the psychiatrist's reaction. The number of people who believe that scientists have proven that depressed people have low serotonin is a glorious testament to the power of market-ing."*

Pfizer is not the only pharmaceutical company to link the "chemical imbalance" theory to the cause of the alleged psychiatric mental illness for which a drug has been approved to treat. In fact, virtually all of the antidepressants reviewed by the FDA for "black box" warnings mention the chemical levels in the brain as possible causes of the alleged mental disorders. The following is a list of what some of the other pharmaceutical companies have to say about the chemical imbalance theory and key words to focus on that provide a glimpse into what really is known by the makers of psychiatric drugs about the alleged mental illnesses the drugs reportedly treat and how the particular drug works on the alleged psychiatric disorders.

While the following explanations are heavy in medical/scientific jargon, what is clear is that none of the pharmaceutical companies know exactly how their drugs work on the reported psychiatric mental illnesses.

Eli Lilly and Co., the makers of the first SSRI antidepressant, Prozac (fluoxetine hydrochloride): "Depression is not fully understood, but a growing amount of evidence supports the view that people with depression may have an imbalance of the brain's neurotransmitters, the chemicals that allow nerve cells in the brain to communicate with each other. Many scientists believe that an imbalance in serotonin, one of these neurotransmitters, may be an important factor in the development and severity of depression. Prozac may help correct this imbalance by increasing the brain's own supply of serotonin." [3] Furthermore, how Prozac works—its clinical pharmacology—is explained by the FDA this way: "The antidepressant, antiobsessive-compulsive, and antibulimic actions of Fluoxetine (Prozac) are presumed to be linked to its inhibition of CNS neuronal uptake of serotonin..." ***Key words: believe, may, presumed.***

Organon Pharmaceutical, the makers of the antidepressant Remeron: "Remeron, introduced by Organon in 1994, is a noradrenergic and selective serotonergic antidepressant (NaSSA), the first of a new class of therapy. Its active compound, mirtazapine, has a dual-action effect aimed at rectifying the chemical imbalances in the brain that are understood to cause depression." [4] The FDA explains Remeron this way: "The mechanism of action of Remeron (mirtazapine) Tablets, as with other drugs effective in the treatment of major depressive disorder, is unknown. Evidence gathered in preclinical studies suggests that mirtazapine enhances central noradrenergic and serotonergic activity..." ***Key words: unknown, suggests.***

Forest Laboratories, Inc., the makers of the antidepressant Lexapro: "As a selective serotonin reuptake inhibitor (SSRI), Lexapro helps restore the brain's chemical balance by increasing the available supply of serotonin, a substance in the brain believed to influence mood." [5] The FDA: "The mechanism of antidepressant action of escitalopram (Lexapro), the S-enantiomer of racemic citalopram, is presumed to be linked to potentiation of serotonergic activity in the central nervous system resulting from its inhibition of CNS neuronal reuptake of serotonin (5-HT)." ***Key words: presumed, believed.***

Wyeth Pharmaceuticals, the makers of antidepressant Effexor: "Effexor XR is known as an SNRI (serotonin and norepinephrine reuptake inhibitor) and is believed to help treat depression and the associated symptoms of anxiety by affecting the level of two chemicals in the brain—serotonin and norepinephrine. These two chemicals are thought to play a key role in depression and the associated symptoms of anxiety. Correcting the imbalance of these two chemicals may help relieve depression symptoms and the associated symptoms of anxiety..." [6] The FDA: "The mechanism of the antidepressant action of venlafaxine in humans is believed to be associated with its potentiation of neurotransmitter activity in the CNS..." ***Key words: believed, thought, and may.***

GlaxoSmithKline, the manufacturer of the antidepressant Wellbutrin: "Research suggests that depression may be caused by an imbalance of brain chemicals called neurotransmitters. Scientists believe that Wellbutrin XL helps balance the levels of two of these neurotransmitters called dopamine and norepinepherine."[7] The FDA: "While the mechanism of action of bupropion, as with other antidepressants, is unknown, it is presumed that this action is mediated by noradrenergic and/or dopaminergic mechanisms." *Key words: suggests, may, believe, unknown, presumed.*

Solvay Pharmaceuticals and Pharmacia & Upjohn jointly market the antidepressant Luvox, GlaxoSmithKline, manufacturer of the antidepressant Paxil, and Forest Laboratories, the manufacturer of the antidepressant Celexa, all report similar "understanding" of their drugs, using similar scientific jargon about how the antidepressants are **"presumed"** to work on the brain chemicals.

While all of the above pharmaceutical companies claim or suggest the particular mind-altering drug either "helps correct," "helps restore," "enhances," or "mediates" the chemical balance in the brain, nowhere on any of the company websites is information provided about any objective, confirmable neurological/biological testing conducted to determine the levels of the alleged "chemical imbalance." All of the above pharmaceutical company websites except Solvay (Luvox) and GlaxoSmithKline (Wellbutrin) offer a "quiz" "checklist" or "self-test" to help determine if an individual may be suffering from one or several of the alleged mental illnesses that the company's drug will "treat."

In other words, the extent of testing for a variety of alleged mental abnormalities, which all of the named pharmaceutical companies either state is due to or suggest may be due to a "chemical imbalance," is as easy as answering questions on a self-test or quiz. Not one of the pharmaceutical company "quiz" questions ask if the would-be patient has had their brain chemical levels evaluated or measured and, if so, what those chemical levels may be.

The above pharmaceutical companies do not understand "completely" how their mind-altering drugs work on the indicated alleged mental illness(s) for which the drugs have been approved for treatment, nor do they provide any objective confirmable evidence of a "chemical imbalance." But the pharmaceutical companies are not alone. In fact, the "chemical imbalance" theory is rampant among private mental health organizations and even in the top echelon of the mental-health experts in the federal government.

For example, the National Alliance for the Mentally Ill (NAMI), which boasts it is "The Nation's Voice on Mental Illness," states, in part, on its website that although "there is no single cause of major depression...whatever the specific causes of depression, scientific research has firmly established that major depression is a biological brain disorder." NAMI then goes on to state "Norepinephrine, serotonin and dopamine are three neurotransmitters (chemical messengers that transmit electrical signals between brain cells) thought to be involved with major depression. Scientists believe that if there is a chemical imbalance in these neurotransmitters, then clinical states of depression result." [8]

To fully appreciate the level of knowledge the "Nation's Voice on Mental Illness" has about the alleged mental disorder depression; one has to take a close look at each part of the organization's explanation of the cause of depression. First, NAMI says "there is no single cause of major depression." Then, having stated that there is no known single cause of depression, NAMI then explains that "scientific research has firmly established that major depression is a biological brain disorder." And, as if to add credence to this definitive statement, NAMI throws in the chemical imbalance theory, "scientists believe that if there is a chemical imbalance in these neurotransmitters, then clinical states of depression result."

One might question that if "scientific research has firmly established that major depression is a biological brain disorder," where is the proof of the objective confirmable biological abnormality? And, if the objective confirmable biological abnormality exists, why does NAMI state up front that "there is no single cause of major depression?" Wouldn't the biology reveal the cause? While the first two parts of the explanation appear to be contradictory, throwing in the "chemical imbalance" theory sounds scientific but only adds to the confusion.

What is clear is that NAMI, in its discussion of depression, does not offer any information to its members about the specific biology that "scientific research has firmly established" and, not unlike the pharmaceutical companies, NAMI also fails to offer information as to where the mental health organization's members may go to have their brain chemicals objectively tested for the alleged chemical imbalances. It is not difficult to understand why NAMI pushes the "chemical imbalance" theory.

According to a December 1999 article in *Mother Jones* magazine by Ken Silverstein titled *Prozac.org: An influential mental health nonprofit finds its 'grassroots' watered by pharmaceutical millions,* the organization received financial support from 18 drug firms, "a total of $11.72 million between 1996 and mid-1999. These include Janssen ($2.08 million), Novartis ($1.87 million), Pfizer ($1.3 million), Abbott Laboratories ($1.24 million), Wyeth-Ayerst Pharmaceuticals ($658,000), and Bristol-Myers Squibb ($613,505)." The leading donor to NAMI was the maker of Prozac, the mother of all pharmacological intervention, pharmaceutical giant Eli Lilly which, according to Silverstein, Lilly "gave $2.87 million during that period." And, perhaps more telling is Silverstein's report that Lilly executive Jerry Radke was "on loan" to NAMI and working out of the organization's headquarters.[9]

The "chemical imbalance" theory has not escaped the intellectual giants of mental health in the federal government but, unlike NAMI and the pharmaceutical industry, on a federal level "chemical imbalance" has not been elevated beyond a theory. A cursory review of the NIMH website offers extensive information about mental illness, including possible causes and treatment of several well-known alleged mental illnesses. For instance, listed under schizophrenia, borderline personality disorder (BPD) and obsessive compulsive disorder, (OCD), the NIMH website discusses the possibility of neurotransmitters and chemicals in the brain interacting as a possible cause of the alleged mental illness. Nowhere, though, does NIMH definitively state that a "chemical imbalance" is the specific cause of any alleged mental illness. In fact, the federal institute makes it clear that while there are many areas being researched to determine the cause of depression and other alleged psychiatric disorders, including chemical levels in the brain, there is no known physiology to identify mental illness.

Although the "chemical imbalance" theory is bandied about as fact by a number of pharmaceutical companies, mental health organizations and an untold number of physicians and psychiatrists, "chemical imbalance" is today, despite decades of research, still a theory and even the NIMH refrains from elevating the theory to the status of medical/scientific fact.

Naturally one wonders how Pfizer got away with the unqualified statement that the company's mind-altering drug/"medicine," Zoloft, **"helps correct the chemical imbalance of serotonin in the brain."** There is a simple answer to this question, and it has nothing to do with objective, confirmable biological or neurological tests and, in fact, whether or not a "chemical imbalance" is the cause of any alleged mental illness isn't even a consideration during the FDA drug approval process.

Peter Breggin, a psychiatrist, court-qualified medical expert, director of the International Center for the Study of Psychiatry and Psychology (ICSPP), and author of more than a dozen books, including *Toxic Psychiatry, Talking Back to Prozac* and *The Anti-Depressant Fact Book,* explains that the FDA couldn't give a hoot about what psychiatric disorder the drugs are alleged to treat. "The pharmaceutical company statements are negligent by FDA standards. The FDA does not approve the drug to correct biochemical imbalance – that has nothing to do with the FDA. The FDA isn't interested in it (the disorder). The FDA approves the drug because, in this case, Pfizer could come up with two studies to show some sort of statistically demonstrable improvement on a couple of parameters (clinical trials). The theory (chemical imbalance) is not what is being tested. What is being tested and considered for approval by the FDA is the clinical efficacy (effectiveness) and adverse effects of the drug being considered. While the FDA may ask for an explanation for why the pharmaceutical company thinks the drug is going to work, the theory of how a drug works has nothing to do with how a drug is approved. Nothing."

"The approval of the drug," says Breggin, "is strictly empirical on the basis of clinical trials showing sufficient efficacy compared to adverse effects. In order to get FDA approval for a drug the pharmaceutical companies conduct clinical trials, and in these trials it is almost always the test where the doctor determines whether the patient feels better that are submitted in support of the approval. If you compare the studies, the vast majority of the time patients do not feel better on these drugs. In clinical trials four or five basic test forms are used. One form will be a patient report; then there are three or four forms where the doctor conducting the clinical trial is simply asking the patient questions, and almost none of the questions are open-ended—there is no opportunity for the patient to say whatever they please. And usually what you see getting improved is eating and sleeping and things that are usually physical. Generally, the questions that are used in clinical trials to get drug approvals are not questions that elicit how a patient feels, but rather observations by the doctor about how the patient is doing, such as questions about appetite, weight loss and sleep patterns, rather than questions like "has your life improved" or "are you feeling better?" The drug company only has to prove that the drug is statistically significantly better than placebo (sugar pill). Usually the outcome is quite marginal and usually most of the studies don't show an improvement over placebo. This fact was made clear during the February 2004 FDA hearings."

Recall that in February and September of 2004, the FDA held hearings to establish whether the SSRI class of drugs was causing self-harm and violent behavior in children. Having reviewed all the available data, the FDA concluded that in 12 of 15 clinical trials the SSRIs under consideration were no more effective than placebo (sugar pills) and acknowledged "an increased risk of suicidal thoughts and behavior ('suicidality') in children and adolescents being treated with antidepressants..." The fact is, according to the FDA review of clinical trial data for the most widely prescribed antidepressants, including Pfizer's Zoloft, the drugs proved no more effective than sugar pills in treating the alleged psychiatric disorder.

A study published by Irving Kirsch (University of Connecticut), Thomas J. Moore (The George Washington University School of Public Health and Health Services) and Alan Scoboria and Sarah S. Nicholls (University of Connecticut), titled *"The Emperor's New Drugs: An Analysis of Antidepressant Medication Data Submitted to the U.S. Food and Drug Administration,"* that analyzed clinical trial data submitted to the FDA to establish the SSRI drugs' efficacy, found that "the pharmacological effects of antidepressants are clinically negligible."[10]

Kirsch et al. cites additional research titled, *"Listening to Prozac but Hearing Placebo: A Meta Analysis of Antidepressant Medication,"* finding that the efficacy data submitted to the FDA for the six most widely prescribed antidepressants approved between 1987 and 1999—fluoxetine (Prozac), paroxetine (Paxil), sertraline (Zoloft), venlafaxine (Effexor), nefazodone (Serzone), and citalopram (Celexa) —showed that 75 percent of the response to the antidepressants is duplicated by placebo.[11] In other words, what the Kirsch team found was that fully three-quarters of the people taking the antidepressants responded as well to the sugar pill as they did to the drug.

In response to commentaries on the "Emperor's New Drugs" study, Kirsch et al. stated that "there is now unanimous agreement among commentators that the mean difference between response to antidepressant drugs and response to inert placebo is very small. It is so small that, despite sample sizes involving hundreds of participants, 57 percent of the trials funded by the pharmaceutical industry failed to show a significant difference between drug and placebo. Most of these negative data were not published (see Thase, 2002) and were accessible only by gaining access to U.S. Food and Drug Administration documents."[12]

The authors further state in "Antidepressants and Placebos" that "the small difference between the drug response and the placebo response has been a "dirty little secret" (Hollon, DeRubeis, Shelton, & Weiss, 2002) known to researchers who conduct clinical trials, FDA reviewers and a small group of critics who analyzed the published data and reached conclusions similar to ours (e.g., Greenberg & Fisher, 1989)…"[13]

The relevance of the above studies and others like them is that the psychiatric mind-altering drugs are approved by the FDA for the treatment of alleged psychiatric disorders that the pharmaceutical companies either definitively state or suggest are due to an alleged "chemical imbalance" in the brain, which to date has never been scientifically or medically proven.

Would it not seem logical to assume that if, in fact, a neurological "chemical imbalance" exists and is the actual cause of an alleged psychiatric disorder, that the results of the "treatment" —the increase of brain chemicals—would be far superior to a sugar pill? In fact, what has recently been revealed in these studies and a host of others is quite the opposite and, worse still, finally, after years of sitting on the fence, the FDA has concluded that the psychiatric mind-altering drugs used in the "treatment" of a growing number of alleged psychiatric mental disorders may cause violent and suicidal behavior.

Joseph Glenmullen, M.D., a clinical instructor in psychiatry at Harvard Medical School and author of several books, including *Prozac Backlash: Overcoming the Dangers of Prozac, Zoloft, Paxil and Other Antidepressants with Safe, Effective Alternatives*, explains some of the failed science into the "chemical imbalance." "One cannot measure serotonin levels in the brain of any patient. Nor can one measure serotonin at specific synapses. Synapses are the spark plugs between nerve cells, junctions where they exchange chemical messages and where drugs are said to work. Blood levels of serotonin are of little use. Not only is blood drawn from an arm far removed from the brain synapse, 95 percent of serotonin in the human body is in the stomach and other tissues, not the brain. Therefore, blood levels of circulating serotonin bear little relation to what is going on in the nervous system. Some studies of the effects of drugs on serotonin are performed on human blood cells, but, again, these cannot provide much of a picture of what is happening in the brain."[14]

"To circumvent these major problems with human subjects," Glenmullen says, "pharmaceutical companies turned to animal models. A rat can be killed and its brain thrown into a blender and mashed to bits. In test tubes, fragments of the smashed brain reconstitute into little spheres, which researchers call synaptosomes, a name evoking synapses in patients, although the ground-up bits of rat brain may have little in common with them. The effect of drugs on serotonin levels in the synaptosomes is measured in test tubes, although the results may bear little relation to the complexity of what the drugs do in the living brain."[15]

Glenmullen concludes, "These test tube studies show Prozac, Zoloft, Paxil and Luvox (SSRI antidepressants) raise serotonin levels. This is where the hypothesis of a serotonin imbalance comes from: extrapolating to humans from test tube studies on blenderized rat brains. Obviously, this is faulty logic, pseudoscience again. This is almost like saying that someone whose headache is relieved by aspirin has an aspirin deficiency. The truth is no one has anything but the vaguest idea of the chemical effects of these drugs on the living human brain."

The Harvard Medical instructor is not alone in his knowledge and scientific assessment of the alleged "chemical imbalance" theory and points to other, well-respected doctors for confirmation. "Thoughtful scientists and clinicians have seriously questioned the concepts of serotonin imbalances, deficiencies, and selectivity. At a 1997 Harvard Medical School conference, Dr. Andrew Nierenberg, director of the depression research program at the Massachusetts General Hospital and a professor at Harvard, reviewed the disease models of depression. Nierenberg explained, "The dark side of all this is that we have many elegant models but the real fact is that [when it comes to] the exact mechanisms by which these things work, *we don't have a clue.*" (italics mine)[16]

Dr. Jerrold Rosenbaum, chairman of the Department of Psychopharmacology at the Massachusetts General Hospital and also a professor at Harvard, agreed: "After all these years, when someone's asked how antidepressants work, the expert answers 'I don't know' and now the people who are less expert are talking about norepinephrine [the form of adrenaline found in the brain] and serotonin." [17]

Glenmullen sums up the extent of known science of the cause of depression and the "chemical imbalance" theory. "What the public has been told in the past decade is truly astounding. While the alleged 'selectivity' of the drugs makes good marketing copy, implying that they target a depression center in the brain, no such center is known to exist. Eventually, scientists may discover real proof that a small percentage of patients have genetically determined, biological symptoms. But we are a long way from any such knowledge. When patients are told otherwise, they are being misled."[18]

Misled? Despite there being not a single conclusive scientific, peer-reviewed article validating a "chemical imbalance" in the brain as the definitive cause of any psychiatric disorder, let alone depression, as has been demonstrated in this chapter, it is nothing but wishful thinking on the part of many in the medical field and pharmaceutical industry. Even the former surgeon general of the

United States, David Satcher, M.D., Ph.D., states: "The diagnosis of mental disorders is **often believed to be more difficult** than diagnosis of somatic (physical), or general medical, disorders, since there is no definitive lesion, laboratory test, or abnormality in brain tissue that can identify the illness." (emphasis mine)[19]

Like APA President Sharfstein, who disingenuously reported in *People* magazine (July 2005) that "We do not have a clean-cut lab test," (for determining a chemical imbalance), knowing full well there is *no* lab test, the former surgeon general is being equally disingenuous in his explanation of diagnosing mental illness. Rather than definitively state that there is "no definitive lesion, laboratory test, or abnormality in brain tissue that can identify the illness," like the pharmaceutical companies that qualify the chemical imbalance with "may" or "believed" to be the cause of depression, Satcher qualifies the statement "diagnosing mental disorders is often believed to be more difficult..."

"Often believed to be?" Is this the best the public can expect from the top minds in mental health, especially in light of the fact that a psychiatric diagnosis can be used to have a person incarcerated in a mental institution? Which is it, sometimes more difficult and sometimes not more difficult? Former surgeon general Satcher's explanation has the same odor as the pharmaceutical companies' statements about how their drugs work: "although the way (drug) works for depression is not *completely* understood," as if there is some real definitive objective understanding about how the mind-altering drugs work in the human brain targeting a specific alleged psychiatric mental illness.

The language chosen by the nation's former top doctor is no accident but, rather, appears to be an attempt to provide reassurance that even though there is not a single solitary definitive objective lab test to diagnose any of the alleged psychiatric mental illnesses—making diagnosis of alleged mental illnesses completely subjective—it is possible to accurately diagnose mental illnesses because it is only "often believed to be more difficult," not always more difficult.

Regardless of the desire of those in medicine and psychiatry to legitimize the "chemical imbalance" theory—the "believed" cause of so many alleged mental disorders—to date there is no scientific evidence to elevate the theory to a bona fide place among known diseases and, however disingenuous, even the former surgeon general was forced to choke up the truth.

Given that no one in medicine is capable of providing the science to support the legitimacy of the chemical imbalance brain abnormality as the cause of any psychiatric disorder, it is not surprising that Pfizer decided to rethink the language the company used to explain how Zoloft works. By August 2005, an entirely new website was launched about Zoloft. Although Pfizer still claims that its mind-altering drug corrects the imbalance of serotonin in the brain, the explanation of how the drug works has gone the way of the other antidepressant manufacturers' language, using the qualifiers "might," "believes" and "could."

The original website language read: "although the way Zoloft works for depression, panic disorder, OCD, and PTSD is not completely understood, *what is understood is that Zoloft is a medicine that helps correct the chemical imbalance of serotonin in the brain.* Serotonin is a naturally occurring chemical in the brain that is involved in the transmission of messages between nerve cells." (italics mine)

The new website language used by Pfizer reads in part: "this tie between depression and serotonin led scientists to an interesting find. Scientists *believe* people with depression *could* have an imbalance of serotonin in their brain. That means the level of serotonin is 'off.' So the nerve cells can't communicate, or send messages to each other the right way. This lack of contact between cells *might* cause depression. Zoloft helps fix this. Zoloft helps the nerve cells send messages to each other the way they normally should."[20] (italics mine)

For years Pfizer publicly stated on the company's website that although the company did not completely understand how its drug worked on the psychiatric disorders for which the drug was approved, the company did understand that Zoloft, "the medicine," "helps correct the chemical imbalance of serotonin in the brain." The company's new website still intimates that it is aware of, or has objective evidence, that a chemical imbalance exists in the brain of those diagnosed with "mental illnesses."

The new language, rather than continue to admit that the company doesn't understand how the drug works on the psychiatric disorders for which it was approved, now provides an explanation about what scientists "believe" "might" be the cause of depression and it "could" be due to an imbalance of serotonin in their brain. But the new language, rather than clarify, raises new questions. For instance, the company now states "that means the level of serotonin is off."

As has been well-documented in this chapter, there are many scientists and doctors who definitively state that a chemical imbalance in the human brain has yet to be proved and there is no known method of measuring the level of chemicals in the living human brain, or what are the accurate levels of chemicals in an individual's brain, one has to wonder how Pfizer knows that any person's serotonin level is "off?"

Furthermore, Pfizer states, "Zoloft helps the nerve cells send messages to each other the way they normally should." Again, what science does Pfizer have to demonstrate what "normal" is in any individual, especially since there is no scientific evidence that proves a chemical imbalance exists in any living human brain?

Despite Pfizer's new qualified language about how Zoloft works, the company continues to make a claim that is scientifically unproven. Recall that the original language stated: "Zoloft is a medicine that helps correct the chemical imbalance of serotonin in the brain." Pfizer still makes this statement, but has qualified it: "*Watch the animation* of how Zoloft works to correct this imbalance of serotonin levels in the brain." (italics mine)

To gain a better understanding of Pfizer's science to support the information provided on the company's website, I wrote to the company's media relations officer asking:

1. Does Zoloft correct the chemical imbalance of Serotonin in the brain? If yes, why not make the statement? If no, what part of the science used to write the first language changed?
2. The new website language states: "that means the level of serotonin is "off." What test is used to determine the level of serotonin is "off?"

3. What test is used to determine the level of serotonin in the brain of a human?

4. What is the correct chemical level in each individual's brain?

5. "Zoloft helps the nerve cells send messages to each other the way they normally should." What does science say is "normal?"

Psychiatrist and court-qualified medical expert, Peter Breggin, who, during an interview about Pfizer's website change, explained that, "Pfizer, for many years on its website, has claimed that Zoloft corrected biochemical imbalances. I've been very critical of that because there is no scientific evidence for it. And they have, I believe, implied it in their television ads. Recently they have corrected, to some extent, their website in regard to removing at least the certainty with which they make these claims. However, through years of making these claims in their advertising and promotional materials, Pfizer helped to create an atmosphere surrounding these drugs, which was misleading and fraudulent and therefore they need to be held responsible for the public's and the profession's mistaken idea that drugs like Zoloft correct biochemical imbalances when, in fact, they (the drugs) create biochemical imbalances of a very severe kind that often have lasting and irreversible effects. They cannot prove a biochemical imbalance exists in the human brain and I suspect they simply will not respond to your questions."

To date, I have received no response to my questions from any representative of Pfizer.

Kelly Patricia O'Meara

[1] Kessler, R., et al, National Comorbidity Survey, June 6, 2005.

[2] Pfizer Pharmaceutical Website "Zoloft" February 2005, http://www.zoloft.com.

[3] Eli Lilly and Company Website "How Prozac Can Help You." http://www.prozac.com.

[4] Organon International Website "Remeron/Mental Health." http://organon.com.

[5] Forest Laboratories, Inc., Website "How Lexapro Works." http"//www.lexapro.com.

[6] Wyeth Pharmaceuticals, Inc. Website " How Effexor XR Works." http://www.effexorxr.com.

[7] GlaxoSmithKline, Website "How Wellbutrin XL Works." http://www.wellbutrin-xl.com.

[8] NAMI Website, "What Are The Causes of Major Depression?" http://www.nami.org.

[9] Ken Silverstein, "Prozac.Org: An influential mental health nonprofit finds its 'grassroots' watered by pharmaceutical millions," *Mother Jones*, Nov/Dec 1999 Issue.

[10] Irving Kirsch, Thomas J. Moore, Alan Scoboria, Sarah S. Nicholls, "The Emperor's New Drugs: An Analysis of Antidepressant Medication Data Submitted to the U.S. Food and Drug Administration," *Prevention & Treatment Volume* 5(1), July 2002, pg-23.

[11] Irving Kirsch, Guy Sapirstein, "Listening to Prozac but Hearing Placebo: A Meta-Analysis of Antidepressant Medication," *Prevention & Treatment* Volume 1(1), June 1998.

[12] Irving Kirsch, Alan Scoboria, Thomas J. Moore, "Antidepressants and Placebos: Secrets, Revelations, and Unanswered Questions," *Prevention & Treatment* Volume 5(1), July 2002.

[13] Ibid.

[14] Glenmullen, Joseph, M.D., "Prozac Backlash: Overcoming the Dangers of Prozac, Zoloft, Paxil and Other Antidepressants with Safe, Effective Alternatives, (Touchstone Books) pg-201

[15] Ibid., pg-202.

[16] Ibid., pg-203.

[17] Ibid., pg-203.

[18] Ibid., pp. 203.

[19] Mental Health: A Report of the Surgeon General, 1999. pp. 44.

[20] Pfizer Pharmaceutical Website "How Zoloft Works" August 2005, http://www.zoloft.com.

Chapter Four

"Kiddie Cocaine"

Wiggling is not acceptable behavior at any age. In fact, wiggling, coupled with not paying attention and even being impulsive all are behavioral "symptoms" that a person is "suffering" from what has become the biggest-selling alleged mental illness among American children and an increasing number of American adults—attention deficit hyperactivity disorder, commonly referred to as ADHD.

The APA's non-scientific manual of alleged mental disorders, the *DSM-IV* (the psychiatric billing bible) provides subjective diagnostic criteria to parents and clinicians to help identify this alleged mental illness so that appropriate treatment/drug recommendations can be made. According to the APA, any six of the following 18 subjective behaviors must be met before a child or adult can be diagnosed with the mental illness, ADHD:

1. *often fails to give close attention to details or makes careless mistakes in schoolwork, work, or other activities*
2. *often has difficulty sustaining attention in tasks or play activities*
3. *often does not seem to listen when spoken to directly*
4. *often does not follow through on instructions and fails to finish schoolwork, chores, or duties in the workplace (not due to oppositional behavior or failure to understand instructions)*
5. *often has difficulty organizing tasks and activities*
6. *often avoids, dislikes, or is reluctant to engage in tasks that require sustained mental effort (such as schoolwork or homework)*

7.   *often loses things necessary for tasks or activities (e.g., toys, school assignments, pencils, books, or tools)*
8.   *is often easily distracted by extraneous stimuli*
9.   *is often forgetful in daily activities*
10.   *often fidgets with hands or feet and squirms in seat*
11.   *often leaves seat in classroom or in other situations in which remaining seated is expected*
12.   *often runs about or climbs excessively in situations in which it is inappropriate (in adolescents or adults, may be limited to subjective feelings of restlessness)*
13.   *often has difficulty playing or engaging in leisure activities quietly*
14.   *is often "on the go" or often acts as if "driven by a motor"*
15.   *often talks excessively*
16.   *often blurts out answers before questions have been completed*
17.   *often has difficulty awaiting turn*
18.   *often interrupts or intrudes on others (e.g., butts into conversations or games).*

These behaviors are symptoms of a mental illness in need of psychiatric treatment? The psycho-wizards seem to think so, but others might argue that they are common behaviors that periodically may or may not positively or negatively affect a person's life that can be subjectively manipulated in order to arrive at a psychiatric diagnosis of mental illness in need of treatment with a mind-altering drug, such as Ritalin. But regardless of how the APA and the psychopharmacology community try to spin it, never in the history of the world, either in life or at autopsy, has an objective, confirmable, biologic or neurologic abnormality been found in the brain, or anywhere else in the body, that proves the existence of the psychiatric mental illness, ADHD.

Despite millions of Americans—including an ever-increasing number of preschool children and toddlers—being diagnosed as suffering from this alleged mental illness, ADHD is just another in the long line of psychiatric diagnoses that cannot be objectively proven. More odd, though, is that it appears that the United States has cornered the market on this particular mental illness. That's right, according to the U.S. Drug Enforcement Administration (DEA), the federal agency responsible for the regulation and control of substances with abuse potential, *"the U.S. produces and consumes 85 percent of the world's methylphenidate, commonly known as Ritalin, one of the mind-altering treatments for the mental illness ADHD."* [1] (italics mine)

This is an astounding factoid and an extraordinary commentary on the deteriorating mental health of America's youth when one considers that ADHD is exclusive to the U.S., and that the remaining 15 percent of consumed methylphenidate is divided among every other nation in the world. But it wasn't always this way. America's children, and later adults, haven't always been considered to be suffering from a mental illness because they wiggled or talked out of turn or any combination of the APA's subjective list of abnormal behaviors.

The switch from normal to abnormal behavior was pulled when in 1987 the deep thinkers at the APA voted to include ADHD in the *DSM-III-R*, which meant treatment for the mental illness could be covered by insurance and quickly escalated the use of mind-altering drugs. The data supports the increase in psychiatric diagnosing when the DEA reported that "prior to 1991, domestic sales reported by the manufacturers of methylphenidate (Ritalin) remained stable at approximately 2,000 kilograms per year." By 1999, however, domestic sales had increased by nearly 500 percent. [2]

The DEA further reports that by 2000, the number of methylphenidate (Ritalin) prescriptions had leveled off at about 11 million per year but, with newer treatments coming into the market, such as Adderall, there was a sharp increase in amphetamine prescriptions for treating ADHD. According to the DEA, "amphetamine prescriptions (primarily Adderall) have increased dramatically since 1996: from about 1.3 million to nearly 6 million between 1996 and 2000. Collectively, this data indicates that the number of prescriptions written for ADHD has increased by a factor of five since 1991."[3]

In other words, the number of children suffering from the exclusive American childhood mental illness ADHD is at what the Centers for Disease Control and Prevention (CDC) would consider an epidemic level. By 2000, approximately 16 million prescriptions were written for either methylphenidate or amphetamine for the alleged mental abnormality ADHD—mind-altering drugs that the DEA and other world health organizations consider to "have the highest abuse potential and dependence profile of all drugs that have medical utility."[4] Methylphenidate (Ritalin and Concerta) and amphetamine (Adderall) are listed by the DEA as Schedule II drugs along with morphine, opium, cocaine and the heroin substitute methadone.

Methylphenidate and amphetamine long have been referred to as "kiddie cocaine" because, according to the DEA, "they produce discriminative stimulus effects similar to cocaine, will substitute for each other and for cocaine in a number of paradigms, and chronic high-dose administration of either drug in animals produces psychomotor stimulant toxicity including weight loss, stereotypic movements and death, and in clinical studies, they produce behavioral, psychological, subjective and reinforcing effects similar to cocaine."[5]

The kicker is the DEA summation: **"this data means that neither animals nor humans can tell the difference between cocaine, amphetamine or methylphenidate when they are administered the same way at comparable doses. In short, they produce effects that are nearly identical."[6]**

Okay, let's recap. Wiggling, talking out of turn and other as sundry behaviors are unacceptable and now abnormal, but millions of American children taking mind-altering drugs that are "nearly identical" to cocaine is acceptable and normal? In other words, chemically altering a child's still developing brain for years on end is okay so long as the desired effect of getting children to sit down and shut up is the end result. Apparently so. And despite the amazing DEA conclusion that American children are daily ingesting the equivalent of cocaine to alter their behavior, the same federal agency says: "Psycho stimulants are effective in treating the symptoms of ADHD."

Call me crazy, but accepting that the DEA knows what it is talking about, one has to wonder why the nation's prisons are full of men and women who have been incarcerated because of cocaine use. What if the incarcerated suffered from the alleged mental illness ADHD and didn't know it (*DSM-IV* "Other (or Unknown) Substance-Related Disorders)" and cocaine was an "effective treatment" of their symptoms? On the other hand, since methylphenidate and amphetamine are "nearly identical" in their effect, and highly addictive, one also has to wonder how many of the incarcerated weren't first introduced to the stimulant Ritalin and then graduated to cocaine because of the psychiatric treatment they received in their youth, which the DEA declares is "effective."

Basic logic begs the question: If methylphenidate and amphetamine are nearly identical to cocaine in their effect, how can the use of one substance be illegal and deserving of jail time and the other "nearly identical" substance legal and considered medicinally helpful? Is this an issue about which entity is legally sanctioned to profit from the mind-altering substance? The other mind-bending thought is: How many mental-health experts—doctors, clinicians and psychiatrists—are diagnosing America's children when they also have been diagnosed with ADHD and are taking this cocaine-like substance as treatment? Put another way, would American parents be comfortable with the family physician if they knew the good doctor had been taking the equivalent of cocaine prior to making the psychiatric diagnosis of their child?

These are not outrageous musings, especially in light of the "Fact Sheet" made available by the DEA about the increasing abuse of methylphenidate:[7]

- Methylphenidate (MPH), most commonly known as Ritalin, ranks in the top 10 most frequently reported controlled pharmaceuticals stolen from licensed handlers.
- Abuse of MPH can lead to marked tolerance and severe psychic dependence.

- Organized drug trafficking groups in a number of states have utilized various schemes to obtain MPH for resale on the illicit market.
- MPH is abused by diverse segments of the population, from health-care professionals and children to street addicts.
- In 1994, a national high school survey (Monitoring the Future) indicated that more seniors in the U.S. abuse Ritalin than are prescribed Ritalin legitimately.
- Students are giving and selling their medication to classmates who are crushing and snorting the powder-like cocaine.

While the DEA's Fact Sheet paints a pretty clear picture of where the drugging of America's youth is heading, it isn't the only organization to raise red flags. In July 2005 the national Center on Addiction and Substance Abuse (CASA) at Columbia University, released a report which details a three-year study of abuse of prescription drugs that would make even the most hardened advocates of the alleged benefits of psychiatric drugs cringe. Joseph A. Califano Jr., CASA's chairman and president and former U.S. secretary of health education and welfare said: "Our nation is in the throes of an epidemic of controlled prescription drug abuse and addiction." The following are just a sample of the results of the CASA study:

- From 1992 to 2002, prescriptions written for controlled drugs increased more than 150 percent, almost 12 times the rate of increase in population and almost three times the rate of increase in prescriptions written for all other drugs.
- From 1992 to 2003, abuse of controlled prescription drugs grew at a rate twice that of marijuana abuse, five times that of cocaine abuse and 60 times that of heroin abuse.
- From 1992 to 2000, the increase in new abusers 12 to 17 years old was far greater than among adults (four times greater for opioids, three times

for tranquilizers and sedatives, and two-and-one-half times for stimulants.

- In 2002 abuse of controlled prescription drugs was implicated in at least 23 percent of drug-related emergency department admissions.

Califano summed up the situation this way "America is in a perfect storm of abuse of mind-altering prescription drugs…" The CASA study and the DEA appear to be on the same page, and despite the DEA's odd admission that psycho-stimulant drugs like Ritalin and Adderall and others (kiddie cocaine) are "effective" in the treatment of the alleged mental illness ADHD, the federal agency also appears to be sending another message – similar to the CASA study conclusions, the drugging of America's youth is out of control.

During a 1996 conference titled "Stimulant Use in the Treatment of ADHD," Deputy Assistant Administrator for the DEA's Office of Diversion Control, Gene Haislip, told the conference (in part): *"These drugs have been overpromoted, overmarketed and oversold. This constitutes a potential health threat to many children and has also created a new source of drug abuse and illicit traffic. The data shows that there has been a 1,000 percent increase in drug abuse injury reports involving methylphenidate for children in the 10-14 age group. This now equals or exceeds reports for the same age group involving cocaine. In some localities as many as 15 to 20 percent of the children have been put on Ritalin or a similar stimulant, [and] there is good reason to conclude that this is "quick-fix," bogus medical practice which is nevertheless producing large profits. We have become the only country in the world where children are prescribed such a vast quantity of stimulants that share virtually the same properties of cocaine."* [8]

While there seems to be little doubt about the similarities between cocaine and the drugs used as treatment for the alleged mental illness ADHD, on the other hand there also seems to be zero understanding of the causes of the mental disorder by the pharmaceutical companies that manufacture the drugs to treat ADHD. Novartis Pharmaceuticals, the makers of Ritalin, provide an extensive website offering pages and pages of information about the alleged mental illness, except what is the known cause—the objective, confirmable abnormality the drug Ritalin supposedly treats.

Novartis explains it this way (in part): "Medical science first reported children with inattentiveness, impulsivity and hyperactivity in 1902. Today ADHD is one of the most common neurobehavioral disorders of childhood and can continue through adolescence and into adulthood. **The causes are currently unknown.**"[9]

One has to wonder what took medical science so long to figure out that children are inattentive, impulsive and hyper. Most parents have recognized this behavior since the beginning of time. Isn't that what children are, always have been and probably always will be? Are these not the very reasons for recess in elementary school, providing time for children to expend their pent-up energy? Conversely, it can be said that there also are parents who worry and are concerned when their children do not exhibit these behaviors. Naturally, the APA has half-a-dozen or more psychiatric mental illnesses to describe these common behaviors, along with their "appropriate" psychiatric treatments/drugs.

Nevertheless, Novartis also admits that how Ritalin works is equally a scientific mystery: "The mode of action in man is not completely understood, but Ritalin presumably activates the brain stem arousal system and cortex to produce its stimulant effect. There is neither specific evidence which clearly establishes the mechanism whereby Ritalin produces its mental and behavioral effects in children, nor conclusive evidence regarding how these effects relate to the condition of the central nervous system."[10] "Not completely understood," "presumably activates" and "no specific or conclusive evidence?"

Again, one has to wonder how many parents were advised by their family physician or psychiatrist, prior to submitting their children to the equivalent of daily doses of cocaine for years on end, that the pharmaceutical company that makes the drug is clueless about how it works in a living brain on the specific alleged mental illness, that essentially it is cocaine and, according to the DEA, the illegal substance, cocaine, would elicit the same behavioral response as the pharmaceutical psychiatric drug. In fact, the medicinal mind-altering drug would elicit the same behavioral response regardless of whether an individual had or had not been diagnosed with ADHD.

Moreover, in the event that Ritalin is *not* working, Novartis has included a section on the company's website that many may construe as the equivalent of a referral to antidepressant use for ADHD: "When stimulant medications do not work or when your child is experiencing depression or anxiety in addition to ADHD, your doctor may prescribe other medications. Antidepressants are not approved by the FDA for treating ADHD, but some doctors have found them useful."[11] This mention is about off-label prescribing of antidepressant drugs – currently the only antidepressant approved by the FDA for ADHD is Eli Lilly's Strattera, which carries with it its own set of potentially life-threatening problems that will be explored later in this and other chapters.

As has been well-demonstrated in Chapter Three of this book, the pharmaceutical manufacturers of the most popular antidepressants, the NIMH and the FDA don't "completely" understand how the mind-altering antidepressants work on other targeted mental illnesses. But like the manufacturers of antidepressants, Novartis isn't the only pharmaceutical company hawking stimulant, cocaine-like treatment, and the others are equally clueless.

Shire Pharmaceuticals produces the treatment Adderall, an amphetamine or speed. According to the company's website for Adderall, **"The exact origin of ADHD is unknown...."**[12] Shire further lists factors such as genetics, abnormal neurotransmitter function (chemical imbalance) and the environment as possibilities of the cause of the mental illness. The FDA explains the clinical pharmacology of Adderall, how it works on the mental illness, like this (in part): "The mode of therapeutic action in Attention Deficit Hyperactivity Disorder (ADHD) *is not known*."[13] (emphasis mine) Then the FDA throws in a line about the chemical imbalance theory to explain what is "thought" to occur in the brain.

In a nutshell, minus all the medical jargon and chemical imbalance yah-yah, neither the pharmaceutical company nor the FDA understand how the drug works to treat ADHD but, hey, it could be due to an imbalance of the naturally occurring chemicals in the brain—and it has been well-demonstrated that this theoretical chemical imbalance abnormality has never been proven.

Moving along to Eli Lilly, the maker of Strattera (atomoxetine), the first non-stimulant drug (antidepressant) approved for treating ADHD, which the company states is a "neurological condition related, in part, to the brain's chemistry and anatomy." This sounds convincing, but what part of thinking – any thinking—isn't part of the brain's chemistry and anatomy? The company's website does not offer a specific section about how Strattera works, but under the "View Press Releases" section, an explanation was provided in a Sept. 29, 2005, Lilly announcement: "Strattera, a Selective Norepinephrine Reuptake Inhibitor, SNRI, is the first FDA-approved non-stimulant to treat ADHD and provide full-symptom relief. It *is not known precisely* how Strattera reduces ADHD symptoms but…"[14] and then the company rambles on about how scientists *believe* the chemicals in the brain blah, blah, blah. (emphasis mine)

The FDA is equally unsure in its description about the way Strattera works: "The precise mechanism by which atomoxetine produces its therapeutic effects in Attention-Deficit/Hyperactivity Disorder (ADHD) *is unknown*…"[15] but it is "thought" to be chemicals, blah, blah, blah. (emphasis mine)

Johnson & Johnson, the makers of the ADHD treatment Concerta (methylphenidate HCl), as explained by its operating company's (McNeil Pharmaceuticals) Concerta website: "ADHD is a real medical condition, recognized and diagnosed in many countries where high-quality scientific studies have been conducted…"[16] Nowhere on the website is information provided about the objective, confirmable abnormality that is ADHD. Rather, lists of the subjective behaviors are provided as proof of the "medical" condition. And, like the other ADHD treatment providers/pharmaceuticals, Johnson & Johnson doesn't specifically know how its drug works in the brain for treating the alleged ADHD and explains: "Many factors can affect the brain and contribute to ADHD symptoms…"[17]

The company moves on to explain the "imbalance in specific brain chemicals," and further adds that ADHD is "highly genetic" and exposure to substances also increases a child's risk of ADHD symptoms. The psychopharmacological crescendo (you knew it was coming) is the company's section called "The Brain and ADHD": "Medications like Concerta(r) help restore brain chemical communications to more normal levels."[18] Ugh!

Again, given that there is no known method of measuring the levels of naturally occurring chemicals in a living brain, making it impossible to know whether the chemicals are in or out of balance, how does the pharmaceutical company know what the "normal" chemical levels in any individual may be?

Curious about what the makers of Concerta believed were "normal levels" of brain chemical communications, and also the method utilized by the company to measure those levels, I contacted McNeil Laboratories, Concerta Medical Center and requested this information. To date, I have received no reply.

Like the makers of Ritalin, Strattera and Adderrall, the makers of Concerta do not know what is "normal," nor do they know exactly how the drugs work in the human brain on the alleged mental illness ADHD and the FDA reinforces this when the federal agency explains the clinical pharmacology: "Methylphenidate HCl is a central nervous system (CNS) stimulant. The mode of therapeutic action in Attention Deficit Hyperactivity Disorder (ADHD) *is not known*. Methylphenidate is thought to...."[19] (emphasis mine) That's right, blah, blah, blah, the drug is *thought* to do something with the brain chemicals.

And, covering all the bases, what does NIMH have to say about the cause of the alleged mental illness ADHD? NIMH provides nearly 20 pages of information about ADHD, and listed under "What Causes ADHD?" NIMH explains: "Scientists are studying causes in an effort to identify better ways to treat, and perhaps someday to prevent, ADHD. They are finding more and more evidence that ADHD does not stem from the home environment, but from biological causes."[20] Then, after listing environmental agents, brain injury, food additives, sugar and genetics, NIMH provides references to studies on the causes of ADHD but provides no conclusive evidence of an objective, confirmable abnormality that is ADHD.

At this point, one has to ask whether a psychopharmacological pattern is developing. Recall that the FDA and the makers of antidepressants do not "completely" understand how the mind-altering drugs work in the treatment of the supposed mental illnesses for which the drugs are marketed. Nor can the FDA or the pharmaceutical companies provide an objective, confirmable abnormality that is any of the psychiatric illnesses.

Put simply, NIMH, the FDA and the pharmaceutical companies have no objective proof of a neurologic/biologic abnormality for any psychiatric diagnosis and, furthermore, neither group of psycho-pharmaceutical wizards know how the drugs work in the brain for treating the psychiatric illness, including ADHD. Regardless of whether the nation's deep thinkers in mental health and the pharmaceutical industry agree that the mental illnesses are real "conditions," "illnesses" and "disorders," consensus does not equate disease. But the "chemical imbalance" theory still is bandied about as if it were a real objective abnormality and the believed cause of most if not all psychiatric mental illnesses.

Fred A. Baughman, M.D., a retired neurologist and author of *The ADHD FRAUD: How Psychiatry Makes "Patients" of Normal Children*, has, for more than a decade, been a leader in the effort to expose the fraud that is ADHD. Having researched, studied and even discovered real diseases, Baughman explains how the scientific/medical community has been complicit with the psycho-pharmaceutical community in perpetrating the fraud: *"As all physicians are taught, must know and are always responsible for determining and imparting honestly to every patient, if no objective abnormality has been found (regardless of symptoms, regardless of psychological/psychiatric findings, opinions, diagnoses) it cannot and must not be said that a disease is present (disease = objective abnormality). Today the abject fraud in which psychiatrists and physicians of many kinds lead the public to believe ADHD and all of the psychiatric diagnoses are actual diseases is the most massive, evil, fraud in medical history."*[21]

Peter Breggin, M.D., founder of the International Center for Study of Psychiatry and Psychology and author of more than a dozen books, including *The Ritalin Fact Book*, *The Antidepressant Fact Book* and *Talking Back to Ritalin*, testified before the Subcommittee on Oversight and Investigations of the House Committee on Education and the Workforce about ADHD: *"Advocates of ADHD and stimulant drugs have claimed that ADHD is associated with changes in the brain. In fact, the NIH [National Institutes of Health] Consensus Development Conference (1998) and the American Academy of Pediatrics (2000) report on ADHD have confirmed that there is no known biological basis for ADHD. Any brain abnormalities in these children are almost certainly caused by prior exposure to psychiatric medication.* "[22]

Breggin is correct in his reporting of the NIH conclusions on ADHD. According to the esteemed group of mental-health experts that gathered in 1998 to discuss ADHD and its treatments, the NIH Consensus Development Conference Statement concluded with 21 clear, concise words: *"Finally, after years of clinical research and experience with ADHD, our knowledge about the cause or causes of ADHD remains speculative."* [23]

Okay, time for another recap. "After years of clinical research and experience" the top dogs in medicine are still speculating? In fact, recall that Novartis, the maker of Ritalin, explained that "scientists first reported" the abnormal behavior in 1902. That means there have been 103 years of experience with and study of this alleged mental illness and still the cause is speculative? In making this "consensus" statement (perhaps not the intent of the conferees) the esteemed panel of experts also debunked the "chemical imbalance" theory as the abnormality that causes ADHD. Chemical imbalance, genetics, environmental factors, parenting and all the other suggested causes that have been pulled out of their... black bags are theories and completely "speculative."

This is madness. In essence, what is happening is that millions of American children are being put on mind-altering drugs—the equivalent of cocaine— everyday and often for years on end, to treat a mental illness that no one can say with certainty an objective, confirmable abnormality even exists? The best and brightest in mental health admit they are speculating—guessing—effectively using America's children as dice in a psychopharmacological crapshoot.

Worse, yet, the psychiatric drugging are carried out under the guise of medical help. Perhaps it's time for a reality check. Imagine for a moment that millions of people (children) are diagnosed with cancer, and this diagnosis (cancer) was voted into existence without any proof of a biological abnormality, and physicians determined the diagnosis by asking the would-be patient questions about their behavior. How many parents would allow a physician to get away with that diagnosis? Furthermore, without objective proof of the abnormality (cancer), how many parents would allow addictive, potentially life-threatening drugs to be administered to their children as treatment, especially in light of the fact that the companies that manufacture the drugs don't understand how the drugs work in the treatment of the cancer? But this is exactly what is happening with the "speculative" mental illness ADHD and every other alleged psychiatric diagnosis, and the mental health community and pharmaceutical companies openly admit it. Still, people want to believe.

Take the nonprofit organization CHADD, Children and Adults with Attention-Deficit Hyperactivity Disorder, which reports a membership of 20,000 with 235 local chapters nationwide. CHADD, an effective lobbying group that reportedly serves individuals with ADHD and their families, receives donations from the pharmaceutical companies that manufacture the drugs used in "treatment" of the mental illness. In 2001-2002 the organization's financial report reflected pharmaceutical support as a little more than 17 percent ($507,000). The organization also reports that it receives 19 percent of its revenue from publications and related educational products and information. The organization did not include under its pharmaceutical support the revenue generated by sales of the organization's *Attention!* magazine by the pharmaceutical companies that then are distributed in doctor's offices. It has been reported and confirmed by CHADD's director of communications that Shire Pharmaceuticals, the makers of Adderall, purchases more than one-half of the copies of the magazine each print run.[24] Furthermore, a large segment of the organization's revenue is provided by the federal government in grants which, along with the pharmaceutical companies support, makes the organization's position on the alleged mental illness understandable. The organization's knowledge of the cause(s) of the mental illness is not.

CHADD's fact sheet on ADHD provides answers about what the organization believes are the causes of the alleged mental illness: "Research clearly indicates that ADHD tends to run in families and that the patterns of transmission are to a large extent genetic. More than 20 genetic studies, in fact, have shown evidence that ADHD is strongly inherited. Yet, ADHD is a complex disorder, which is undoubtedly the result of multiple interacting genes. Other causal factors (such as low birth weight, prenatal maternal smoking and additional prenatal problems) may contribute to other cases of ADHD. Problems in parenting or parenting styles may make ADHD better or worse, but these do not cause the disorder. ADHD is clearly a brain-based disorder. Currently research is under way to better define the areas and pathways that are involved."[25]

Huh? Where does one begin to wade through this psycho-babble yah, yah? In a nutshell, CHADD is as clueless as the NIH, the APA and the pharmaceutical companies when it comes to the cause(s) of ADHD. Rather than take the time to dissect CHADD's explanation of the believed causes of ADHD, it is much more enlightening and practical to simply refer back to the very direct 21 words of the expert NIH Consensus Statement: "Finally, after years of clinical research and experience with ADHD, our knowledge about the cause or causes of ADHD remains speculative."

Now that it has been established that no one knows the cause or causes, or how the mind-altering drugs work in the brain for the treatment of the alleged mental illness ADHD, one might begin to ask: What is known? Although the drug companies don't know how the drugs work as treatment and are not required to prove the "mechanism" of action, they are required to conduct short-term clinical trials in order to receive FDA drug approval. The pharmaceutical companies must prove that the drug is safe and effective and they must provide to the FDA data supporting that safety and efficacy and also whether there are any adverse effects associated with the mind-altering drugs.

First, though, it is important to remember that the DEA has, in no uncertain terms, equated the usage of methylphenidate and amphetamine with cocaine—"nearly identical in their effect." And, of course, most Americans are familiar with the "this is your brain, this is your brain on drugs" television public-service announcement, referring to those illicit and illegal drugs that do bad things to your child's brain. The following is a partial list of what the 2005 *Physicians' Desk Reference* (*PDR*) report as adverse reactions to the "medicinal" pharmaceutical drugs used as "treatment" for ADHD. (in part)

Ritalin (methylphenidate):
- Nervousness, insomnia, hypersensitivity, anorexia, nausea, dizziness, palpitations, headache, dyskinesia, drowsiness, blood pressure and pulse changes, tachycardia, angina, cardiac arrhythmia, abdominal pain, toxic psychosis, abnormal liver function and weight loss.

Adderall (amphetamine):
- Palpitations, tachycardia, psychotic episodes at recommended doses (rare), overstimulation, restlessness, dizziness, insomnia, tremor, restlessness, diarrhea, anorexia, impotence, dyskinesia, and tremor.

Concerta (methylphenidate HCl):
- Blurred vision, abnormal liver function, palpitations, arrhythmia, nervousness, hypersensitivity, dizziness, headache, blood pressure and pulse change, tachycardia, angina, abdominal pain, hepatic coma and insomnia.

Strattera (atomoxetine):
- Palpitations, dizziness, insomnia, headache, fatigue, mood swings, sexual dysfunction, impotence, menstrual disorder, sleep disorder, vomiting, abdominal pain, irritability.

After reviewing the above possible adverse reactions associated with these psychiatric drugs, many may rightfully question how the alleged benefit outweighs the known risk. And although many would consider the above adverse reactions enough information to "Just Say No" to the medicinal help, there may be other possible, and perhaps, more startling, life-threatening consequences associated with the treatment of the alleged mental illness ADHD, including cancer.

In January 1996 the National Toxicological Program of the U.S. Department of Health and Human Services (HHS) released it findings of a two-year carcinogenicity study on methylphenidate, where adult rats and mice were fed Ritalin over a two-year period. The results showed that the mice developed "a statistically significant incidence of liver abnormalities and tumors, including highly aggressive rare cancers known as hepatoblastomas."[26] None of the rats in the study developed abnormalities, and it is this fact that apparently prompted the FDA to continue its support of the psychiatric drug: "FDA considers the results of the studies a signal of a weak cancer-causing potential for this drug—the positive findings were seen in only one organ (the liver) which is known to be particularly likely to develop tumors to a wide variety of stimuli and there was no increase in mortality associated with the tumors." Great! The cancer only showed up in one organ, only in mice, not rats, and none of the rodents died.

Despite the FDA's upbeat response to the study the drug approval agency did, however, ask the drug's sponsor to include the positive findings in the labeling for Ritalin, and to alert prescribers to the "weak signal" by sending them a "Dear Doctor" letter. The FDA further suggested that additional studies were needed.

Samuel S. Epstein, M.D., chairman of the Chicago-based Cancer Prevention Coalition responded to the FDA and the American Academy of Pediatrics support of continued Ritalin use in a Oct. 4, 2001, letter (in part): *"concerns on Ritalin's cancer risk are more acute in view of the millions of children treated annually with the drug and the escalating incidence of childhood cancer, by some 35 percent over the last few decades, quite apart from delayed risks of cancer in adult life. There is no justification for prescribing Ritalin, even by highly qualified pediatricians and psychiatrists, unless parents have been explicitly informed of the drug's cancer risks. Otherwise, prescribing Ritalin constitutes unarguable medical malpractice."*[27]

In February 2005 the results of another study on methylphenidate (addressing chromosome damage) was reported by researchers at the University of Texas Medical Branch at Galveston and the University of Texas M.D. Anderson Cancer Center in Houston. The Texas researchers drew and tested blood from 12 children diagnosed with ADHD prior to methylphenidate treatment. After having taken standard therapeutic doses of methylphenidate for three months, the children's blood was again drawn and tested and researchers found a threefold increase in levels of chromosome abnormalities—occurrences associated with increased risks of cancer and other adverse health effects. One of the lead researchers, Randa A. El-Zein, M.D., Ph.D., said most of the abnormalities found in the studied blood cells consisted of chromosome breaks "and a higher frequency of aberrations is reported to be associated with an increased risk of cancer down the line. It was pretty surprising that all of the children taking methylphenidate showed an increase in chromosome abnormalities in a relatively short period of time."[28]

Although the results appear to be in the same ballpark as the 1995 rodent study, the Texas researchers acknowledge that there is much still unknown about methylphenidate and cancer. The authors of the study admit that the sample size was small and that much larger tests are needed, including finding answers to such questions as: Do the levels of chromosome abnormalities return to normal when patients stop taking methylphenidate? Only further testing will answer such an important question, but one has to wonder how many physicians even are aware of these important studies, and also how many parents are routinely advised about the studies when methylphenidate is recommended as treatment for the alleged mental disorder.

Furthermore, if the DEA is correct and there are an estimated 11 million prescriptions written yearly for the mind-altering cocaine-like methylphenidate, one also has to be concerned that the available pool of children *not* being or having been treated with methylphenidate or a number of other mind-altering treatments is becoming more and more limited and, subsequently, finding "clean" study participants will become increasingly difficult.

Despite millions of Americans daily using the mind-altering drug for years on end, there are very few long-term studies on the safety and efficacy of methylphenidate. This is backed up by a 2005 study conducted by the Oregon State University Drug Effectiveness Review Project (ODER). Researchers analyzed 2,287 studies done on drugs used as treatment for ADHD and found no evidence on long-term safety of drugs to treat ADHD in young children or adolescents; safety evidence is of poor quality; evidence that ADHD drugs help adults is not compelling; the way the drugs work is not well understood; there are no trials of comparative effectiveness of these drugs for treatment of ADHD; good quality evidence is lacking on the use of drugs to affect outcomes relating to global academic performance, consequences of risky behaviors, social achievements, etc. [29]

The ODER report reinforces the same line that came out of the mental health experts at the NIH after the 1998 conference on ADHD—nobody knows anything, zero, zip, nada, a big hole in a donut, about the cause of ADHD. No conclusive evidence of what causes the alleged mental illness, no conclusive evidence of how the drugs manufactured to treat the alleged mental illness actually work in the brain, no conclusive evidence about long-term safety, no conclusive evidence about the effectiveness of the drugs to treat the alleged mental illness. Remember the experts said it best: they are just "speculating." Is it any wonder that this examination, another in a long line of studies, came to the same conclusions?

While the supposed benefits of ADHD treatments remain "speculative" at best, what is coming to light is that government health agencies here and around the world finally are taking notice of some of the adverse effects of some of the mind-altering drugs marketed for the treatment of the alleged psychiatric disorder. Recall that in 2003 the British equivalent of the FDA effectively banned the use of antidepressants in children. This was followed up in October 2004 when the FDA "requested" black box warnings be added to the labels of antidepressants for prescribing to the adolescent population in the U.S. because of a risk of suicidal ideation.

In February 2005, Health Canada, the Canadian equivalent of the FDA, announced that it was withdrawing the ADHD "treatment" Adderall from its market due to "safety information concerning the association of sudden deaths, heart-related deaths and strokes in children and adults taking the usual recommended doses of Adderall and Adderall XR."[30] The FDA followed up the Canadian decision by releasing a Feb. 9, 2005, "Statement on Adderall," which effectively referred to the Canadian decision to withdraw the drug, but added the "FDA does not feel that any immediate changes are warranted in the FDA labeling or approved use of this drug based upon its preliminary understanding of Health Canada's analyses of adverse event reports…"[31]

The FDA further reported in a Feb. 9, 2005, "Public Health Advisory" that "because it appeared that patients with underlying heart defects might be at increased risk for sudden death, the labeling for Adderall XR was changed in August 2004 to include a warning that these patients might be at particular risk, and that these patients should ordinarily not be treated with Adderall products."[32]

What is interesting about the FDA's "Public Health Advisory" is that the 2005 *PDR* already provided a section under "ADVERSE REACTIONS" for Adderall that lists a number of cardiovascular adverse reactions: Palpitations, tachycardia (excessively rapid heartbeat) and elevation of blood pressure. The *PDR* further reports "there have been isolated reports of cardiomyopathy (a serious heart disease in which the heart muscle becomes inflamed) associated with chronic (long-term) amphetamine use."

It would appear that the medical field and the FDA had at their disposal information about the "isolated reports" of cardiovascular problems associated with this drug prior to the Canadian and FDA alerts. Still, one has to wonder how many children are given a complete medical work-up, including cardiovascular tests, before ADHD treatment is prescribed. Then, again, perhaps these "isolated reports" only are important to those few families who experienced one of the particular cardiovascular adverse reactions, like the sudden death of their child. Despite the concerns surrounding the adverse effects of the ADHD "treatment," Canadian authorities lifted the Adderall XR suspension six months later.

Another ADHD treatment hit the news when on Sept. 29, 2005; the FDA announced that it had directed the maker of Strattera, Eli Lilly, to revise its labeling and boxed warning on the mind-altering drug to "alert health care providers to an increased risk of suicidal thinking in children and adolescents." This is an especially interesting "Public Health Advisory" because the alleged mental illness, ADHD, is *not* associated with suicidal thoughts (recall the long list of symptoms at the beginning of the chapter) so one might rightly conclude that the "increased risk" is caused by Strattera. In fact, the FDA determined that one of the points that needed to be included in the "black box" warning: "Strattera increases the risk of suicidal thinking in children and adolescents with ADHD."

But Lilly's "increased risk of suicide" isn't the first trip to the FDA woodshed for Strattera. An earlier FDA Talk Paper titled "New Warning for Strattera," issued in December 2004, requested Eli Lilly to update the label with a warning about the potential for severe liver injury. The FDA label request warns that "severe liver injury may progress to liver failure resulting in death or the need for a liver transplant in a small percentage of patients."

Okay, let's recap once more. Strattera may increase the risk of suicide *and* cause liver problems that could result in death? How bad must the wiggling, talking out of turn and losing homework be that a parent would decide the alleged benefit of taking Strattera, or any of the mind-altering drugs manufactured to treat ADHD, outweighed the known risk of the serious and potentially life-threatening side effects?

Before addressing that question, one must also consider another problem associated with treating children with antidepressants and the equivalent of cocaine daily for years on end—the possible peripheral effect. That's right, recall that *insomnia* is listed as an adverse reaction for methylphenidate and amphetamine and even the antidepressant, Strattera. In October 2005, Medco Health Solutions (a pharmacy/prescription tracking service) announced that children between the ages of 10 and 19 using sleep aids (prescription drugs) increased 223 percent from just five years earlier. Medco determined that from the first six months of 2004, 15 percent of the children using sleep aids also were being treated for ADHD. Medco could not determine whether the alleged disorder or the medication used in treatment was causing the sleep problems.[33]

Let's see, insomnia is a reported adverse reaction in every one of the "medications" used in the "treatment" of ADHD, but no one can be sure what is causing kids to need sleep medication? Why should anyone be surprised by this conclusion? No one in mental-health officialdom knows anything about what causes ADHD or even how the drugs work in the individual brain for treating ADHD.

In the end, it is difficult to know how much of this important information is actually known by the family physicians that now are the lead prescribers of these drugs, and then how much of that information is passed on to parents, but one can be sure of a few things. First, according to the psychiatric/mental-health experts, there is no proof available today of an objective, confirmable abnormality that is the alleged mental illness ADHD—that the diagnosis is purely subjective and "speculative" and, secondly, the pharmaceutical companies that manufacture the mind-altering treatments openly admit they do not understand how the drugs work in the living brain for the stated alleged mental illness. Furthermore, the DEA has made it clear that the drugs used in the treatment of ADHD, except Eli Lilly's antidepressant Strattera, are nearly identical to cocaine in their effect.

Finally, the FDA has officially warned the public about the known possible risks associated with the mind-altering treatments, so it is up to each parent to decide whether the yet-to-be confirmed benefits outweigh the known risks. Despite the fact that the FDA has approved the drugs for treatment of the alleged mental illness, the federal drug agency also has made it clear that the decision to use the psychiatric mind-altering drugs could be a life or death decision. In what can only be described as a psychopharmacological crapshoot, parents are being forced to ask themselves if they're feeling lucky with their child's life.

[1] Terrence Woodworth, Deputy Director, Office of Diversion Control, Drug Enforcement Administration "DEA Congressional Testimony" Committee on Education and the Workforce: Subcommittee on Early Childhood, Youth and Families, May 16, 2000

[2] Ibid.

[3] Ibid.

[4] Ibid.

[5] Ibid.

[6] Ibid.

[7] Drug Enforcement Administration, "Fact Sheet" Methylphenidate, October 20, 1995, http://www.dea.gov.

[8] Gene R. Haislip, "Statement of Drug Enforcement Administration" Conference on Stimulant Use in the Treatment of ADHD, San Antonio, Tx., December 10-12, 1996

[9] Novartis Pharmaceuticals website, An Overview of ADHD. http://www.adhdinfo.com.

[10] Novartis Pharmaceuticals Website "Clinical Pharmacology."

[11] Novartis Pharmaceuticals Website "Antidepressant Medications."

[12] Shire Pharmaceuticals Website AdderallXR "Causes of ADHD," http://www.adderallxr.com.

[13] Food and Drug Administration Website "Clinical Pharmacology" AdderallXR.

[14] "Lilly Announces Important Strattera Label Update" September 29, 2005, Lilly Strattera Website, http://newsroom.lilly.com.

[15] Food and Drug Administration Website "Clinical Pharmacology" Strattera, http://www.fda.gov.

[16] McNeil Consumer & Specialty Pharmaceuticals, "Concerta" Website "Science Made Simple," http://www.concerta.net.

[17] Ibid.

[18] Ibid.

[19] Food and Drug Administration, Clinical Pharmacology, Concerta.

[20] National Institute of Mental Health Website, Attention Deficit Hyperactivity Disorder, http://www.nimh.nih.gov.

[21] Fred A. Baughman, Jr., M.D., January 23, 2005.

[22] Peter R. Breggin, M.D., Testimony Subcommittee on Oversight and Investigations Committee on Education and the Workforce,

[23] Diagnosis and Treatment of Attention Deficit Hyperactivity Disorder. NIH Consensus Development Conference Statement, November 16-18, 1998

[24] Kelly Hearn, *AlterNet* "Here, Kiddie, Kiddie," November 29, 2004.

[25] CHADD, "Fact Sheet #1 The Disorder Named ADHD, CHADD Website, http://www.chadd.org.

[26] Campaignfortruth website "Ritalin and Cancer?"

[27] Samuel S. Epstein, M.D., Cancer Prevention Coalition "Ritalin and Liver Cancer," http://preventcancer.com.

[28] Randa A. El-Zein, M.D., Ph.D., Study Shows Methylphenidate Linked to Chromosomal Changes.

[29] Oregon State University, Drug Effectiveness Project "Pharmacologic Treatments for ADHD," September 2005, Pg- 13-21.

[30] Health Canada, "Advisory" "Health Canada Suspends the market authorization of Adderall XR, a drug prescribed for Attention Deficit Hyperactivity Disorder (ADHD) in children." February, 9, 2005.

[31] U.S. Food and Drug Administration, "Statement on Adderall" February 9, 2005.

[32] U.S. Food and Drug Administration, "Public Health Advisory for Adderall and Adderall XR," February 9, 2005

[33] Reuters, "Prescription Sleep Aid Use for Younger Americans," October 17, 2005

Chapter Five

School Shooters:
Were they doped into killing?

Jeff Weise joined the ranks of dozens of American "school shooters" when on March 21, 2005, the 16-year-old, armed with his grandfather's police-issued shotgun and semiautomatic pistol, shot and killed five students, a teacher and a school security guard. Seven others were wounded. Before going on his shooting rampage at Red Lake High School on the Red Lake Indian Reservation in Northern Minnesota, Weiss fired 13 shots in the home of his grandfather, killing him and his grandfather's girlfriend. The carnage ended a short time later when Weiss took his own life in the same classroom where six of his victims lay dead.

In less than 10 minutes, and with 45 gunshots, the Red Lake assault became the second-deadliest school shooting in U.S. history and, at the end of the day, 10 people, including the shooter, were dead, seven others wounded and a nation watched in horror, again wondering why. The best and brightest in mental health, education and law enforcement have been contemplating this question for more than a decade, unable to come to meaningful conclusions. While officialdom may never completely understand the reasons behind a child's inexplicable and indiscriminate decision to brutally kill classmates and loved ones, one could confidently bet the family farm that the answers will never be found until all the elements are seriously considered.

In the aftermath of the Red Lake school shootings, a *New York Times* article quotes Tammy Lussier, Weise's aunt, "They kept upping the dose for him, and by the end he was taking three of the 20-milligram pills a day. I can't help but think it was too much, that it must have set him off." Lee Cook, another relative of Weise's, said in the same article, "I do wonder on top of everything else he had going on in his life, on top of all the other problems, whether the drugs could have been the final straw." [1]

Were these the hysterical musings of relatives looking for an easy answer—any answer—to rationalize the troubled teenager's horrific actions, or had Weise's bewildered family raised an important question that, in spite of the fact that prescription psychiatric drugs have been involved in a growing number of the recent spate of school shootings, remains inexplicably taboo.

According to news accounts, Weise suffered from depression, had been hospitalized for suicidal tendencies and, sometime in the summer prior to the attack, had been prescribed the antidepressant Prozac. During that time, according to his relatives, the prescription had been increased on at least one occasion, and it was reported that he was taking up to 60 milligrams per day of the mind-altering drug. What is unknown is whether Weise earlier had been diagnosed with another alleged mental illness, such as ADHD, and when exactly was his first encounter with psychiatric help? Is it possible that he had been prescribed other mind-altering drugs prior to his introduction to Prozac? And, worse yet, had he been taking a cocktail (more than one) of prescription psychiatric drugs?

These are important questions that may assist investigators in understanding why children flip out and turn into murderers, but they also are questions rarely asked and apparently deemed unimportant by investigators. Making matters worse, because the majority of school shooters are minors, health records (including mental health data) are sealed by the courts, leaving the public at the mercy of news reports that rely on regurgitations of gossip, rumor and opinion. Often what is known, or what is released to the public about the adolescent's mental health state, is as oblique as "the shooter had been receiving psychiatric help." That is not much to go on and, for most Americans, this statement hardly would register as significant on this-is-important-information-radar, but for those who closely watch the issue; the mere mention of "psychiatric help" is becoming a red flag that psychiatric mind-altering drugs are involved.

While it seems impossible for anyone to possess the ability to fully explain the mysteries of the mind that lead to such murderous rage, in order to gain some understanding of why children kill it nevertheless seems appropriate and even necessary that investigators would consider it important to look at the child's state of mind prior to and at the time of the killings. It is immensely helpful to know that there is no science to support a single psychiatric diagnosis, insomuch as there is no objective, confirmable abnormality to support the psychiatric label, and also that the FDA officially has warned the public that antidepressants and other psychiatric drugs may cause violent and suicidal behavior. So, it would seem important to possess some basic knowledge about how the mind-altering drug Prozac could adversely affect Weise, which might shed some light on his state of mind at the time of the shooting.

The 2005 *Physicians' Desk Reference* (*PDR*) lists the following as some of the known adverse reactions to pharmaceutical giant Eli Lilly's Prozac (fluoxetine HCl); *anxiety, insomnia, agitation, amnesia, confusion, depression, depersonalization, hallucinations, hostility, paranoid reaction, psychosis, delusions, neurosis, malaise, suicide attempt, acute brain syndrome, antisocial reaction, mania, hypomania and akathisia (a feeling of inner physical and emotional torment).*[2]

The *PDR* further informs that "because Prozac may impair judgment, thinking or motor skills, patients should be advised to avoid driving a car or operating hazardous machinery until they are reasonably certain that their performance is not affected."[3] One can only wonder whether, and to what extent, Prozac "impaired" Weise at the time of the shooting. The PDR provides further information that may provide a better understanding of Weise's level of impairment. According to the *PDR*, treatment of Prozac in children and adolescents "should be initiated with a dose of 10 or 20 mg/day. After one week at 10 mg/day, the dose should be increased to 20 mg/day. However, due to higher plasma levels in lower-weight children, the starting and target dose in this group may be 10 mg/day. A dose increase to 20 mg/day may be considered after several weeks if insufficient clinical improvement is observed."[4] This is the prescribing information Eli Lilly thought appropriate for children's use of Prozac, yet 16-year-old Weise reportedly had been prescribed and was taking 60 mg/day.

So that's how it works. The kid isn't better at 10 milligrams, then let's up the mind-altering drug dosage to 20 milligrams. Darn, 20 milligrams don't work, how about 40 or even 60? Still not working, hey, why not 160!

Or, maybe, the truth is that the boy was being treated for an alleged psychiatric mental disorder that is not based in science (an objective, confirmable abnormality of the brain) and was prescribed a mind-altering drug—in dosages that many would consider adult levels—which the pharmaceutical company openly admits it does not understand how the drug works in the human brain for the stated psychiatric diagnosis. Worse still, the mind-altering drug can *cause* the very behavior it is alleged to treat. Maybe Weise was another of the unlucky number of people who experienced psychologically devastating adverse reactions to the mind-altering drugs that the FDA warns about.

But this is not something most mental-health experts will eagerly admit. No, what the deep thinkers in psychiatry continually fall back on is the old stand-by, the psychiatric ace in the hole: "Well, he had a mental illness." Despite zero proof that any psychiatric mental disorder is an abnormality of the brain, the psycho wizards get away with this conclusion because objective, confirmable proof of the alleged brain abnormality is not now, nor has it ever been, demanded or even debated by policymakers.

Mental-health officialdom *says* Weise was mentally ill, so the 16-year-old *must* have been mentally ill, end of discussion. The drugs could not possibly be what triggered the deadly shooting spree. Even though the pharmaceutical company makes it known that the adverse reactions to the drug include depression, mania, hostility, hallucinations and a host of other violent, troubling behaviors, it is the unknown phantom mental illness that is responsible, not the adverse reactions to the drug.

In a July 2005 FDA Alert the agency warned: **"Children taking antidepressants may increase suicidal thoughts and actions in about 1 out of 50 people[age] 18 years or younger. The FDA has approved fluoxetine (Prozac) for treating children who have depression or obsessive-compulsive disorder."**[5] Prozac patient Weise, committed suicide after killing nine other schoolmates, school officials and loved ones. What is more telling, however, is that the makers of Prozac apparently are confused about adolescent treatment with Prozac.

Although Prozac had been approved by the FDA in January 2003 for use in adolescents, one year later, in December 2003, Eli Lilly issued a letter to physicians in the United Kingdom, which states that Prozac is **"not recommended"** for children. Why not? The chemical structure of the mind-altering drug is the same overseas as it is in the United States, so if it's okay for American children, why is it not recommended for British children? Certainly the chemical make-up of the brain is no different with British children than American children. The answer may lie in the fact that the United Kingdom has taken a hard line on the prescribing of antidepressant mind-altering drugs and have effectively banned the use of them on children.

Okay, time for a reality check. Prozac is not recommended for children in the United Kingdom but it is okay for American children. Yeah, that makes sense! The fact is that millions of American children daily take antidepressants, including Prozac, so one has to seriously wonder: Was Weise the "1 out of the 50" that the FDA warned about? If the motive for the shooting rests on evidence (if only for the mere fact that violent behavior is a documented adverse reaction of psychiatric antidepressant drugs) would not investigation 101 dictate at least a discussion about the mind-altering drugs? Given the FDA warnings, one might logically conclude that gathering information about psychiatric drug use by the perpetrator(s) would be a normal part of any investigation.

In reality, what becomes clear as one works through the list of the more famous school shootings over the last 10 years, the prescribed drugs rarely are even a consideration. Worse yet, whether a child-shooter has been prescribed a mind-altering psychiatric drug is only made public if the information is leaked by friends or family. Eric Harris and Dylan Klebold, who went on a murderous assault at Columbine High School in Littleton, Colo., are perfect examples of leaked and protected information about psychiatric drug use.

When it comes to school shooting tragedies, the attack at Columbine is the granddaddy of all child-perpetrated assaults. Eighteen-year-old Harris and 17-year-old Klebold planned and executed the grisliest, most inhumane and senseless schoolhouse attack the nation had ever known. The teenagers savagely had exposed our vulnerabilities and, together, we mourned the innocent victims. TV coverage of the unfolding event brought the assault into seemingly safe and insulated family rooms, planting the seed of fear and in effect putting every mother and father on notice that the unthinkable, a parent's worst nightmare, is more than a remote possibility.

So what is known about the two boys who so brutally extinguished the lives of a dozen classmates and a teacher, and left 24 others seriously wounded, before killing themselves? Despite one of the most intensive investigations of any school shooting, the public still has not been provided all the pieces to the puzzle. The basic information about the shooters provides little in the way of clues to their murderous madness. Harris and Klebold came from two-parent, middle-class, suburban homes, both having played little-league baseball. Harris reportedly had been a Boy Scout. Contrary to reportage, neither of the shooters were members of the "Trenchcoat Mafia" or practicing members of the "Goth" scene.

According to extensive information provided in the Jefferson County, Colo., Juvenile Diversion Program files, it appears that the downward spiral began 13 months prior to the assault when both boys found themselves on the wrong side of the law for having broken into a van and stealing property. Harris and Klebold were charged with criminal trespassing, theft and criminal mischief and offered a diversion program, including 12 months of intervention, counseling and community service.

Harris was directed to attend anger management classes and, at his parent's request, began receiving psychiatric therapy, which included prescribing the then 17-year-old the mind-altering psychiatric drugs Zoloft and Luvox. Both boys excelled in intervention and were released early from the program.

It apparently was during this same time that the would-be shooters maintained a website openly demonstrating intended violence, posting such remarks as "God, I can't wait until I can kill you people," and "I'll just go to some downtown area in some big ass city and blow up and shoot everything I can."[6] It also was during this time that the two were experimenting with homemade pipe bombs and even posting results of explosions on their website. Finally, having illegally obtained an arsenal of weapons and ammunition from a number of sources, on April 20, 1999, Harris and Klebold committed premeditated, cold-blooded, mass murder.

On the surface, the teenagers appear to come from stable, loving homes in which the parents were actively engaged in their lives. The 1998 arrest was a first criminal offense for the pair, and the two seemingly had mended their troubled ways. In fact, according to the Juvenile Diversion Program file, the soon-to-be mass murderers were well on their way to happy normal lives. Although it still is unclear whether Klebold was under the influence of prescribed psychiatric drugs, there is no documentation in Klebold's diversion file to suggest that he was receiving any psychiatric counseling or taking any psychiatric drugs before or at the time of the shooting rampage. And, Klebold had so successfully completed the diversion program that his diversion officer, Robert Kriegshauser, had this to say: "Dylan is a bright young man who has a great deal of potential. If he is able to tap his potential and become self-motivated he should do well in life. Dylan has earned the right for an early termination. He needs to strive to self-motivate himself so he can remain on a positive path. He is intelligent enough to make any dream a reality, but he needs to understand hard work is part of it."[7]

Another entry in Klebold's diversion file, which is undated and the author is unknown states: "nice young man, kind of goofy, and a bizarre sense of humor. He makes me laugh."[8] Despite having been evaluated by a mental-health professional, Klebold had not been diagnosed as suffering from any alleged psychiatric mental disorder and by all accounts of those involved in Klebold's restitution, he was "nice," "funny," "intelligent" and "motivated." Klebold's autopsy results have never been made public, making it difficult to know with any certainty if or what drugs were in his system at the time of the murders.

The file of Klebold's partner in crime, Eric Harris, provides details that for unknown reasons have been missed or deemed insignificant, but, nevertheless, are pieces of the puzzle that many might consider important. According to Harris' diversion program file, the 17-year-old began receiving psychiatric counseling and taking the antidepressant Zoloft for depression in February 1998. An unknown diversion officer for Harris notes in mid-April 1998 that "Eric has been having difficulty with his medication for depression. A few nights ago he was unable to concentrate and felt restless. He went to the Dr. [and] is changing his medication. He can't start the new medication for 2 weeks b/c the Zoloft needs to get out of his system first. He is a little concerned about how he will feel for the next two weeks."[9] What is significant about Harris being prescribed the mind-altering drug is that the FDA has not approved the use of Zoloft for "depression" in adolescents.

Two weeks later, the same unknown diversion officer writes, "Eric is feeling okay now that he isn't on medication, but knows he will feel better when he begins his new medication." And in mid-May 1998 Harris' diversion officer reports that he "began new medication, doesn't feel a difference yet. His Dr. said it would take a few weeks," and during Harris' mid-June session the unknown author writes "medication is good, he is controlling his stress well." [10]

Finally, in mid-July 1998, the unknown author writes that Harris "reports that his medication dosage is changing and he will be taking 100mg now. The unknown diversion officer closes his file on Harris saying, "Really nice young man. Seems responsible and remorseful. He suffers from depression, he changed meds and feels better, he has difficulties handleing (sic) stress, but says he has a good handle on it now. I am not at all worried about drug use from Eric; pretty good head on shoulders (now watch he will get a hot UA [positive urine analysis] for Acid or something)."[11] Diversion officer Robert Kriegshauser wrote the "Termination Report" on Harris saying, "Prognosis: Good. Eric is a very bright young man who is likely to succeed in life. He is intelligent enough to achieve lofty goals as long as he stays on task and remains motivated. Eric should seek out more education at higher levels. He impressed me as being very articulate and intelligent. These are skills that he should grow and use as frequently as possible." [12]

Again, as in the case of Klebold, Harris apparently wowed the law enforcement counselors and sailed through the diversion program with glowing accolades and, yet, two months later the seemingly healthy, intelligent, mentally sound, "likely to succeed" boys had planned and intended to wipe out an entire high school population. The troubling aspect of Harris' file is that the diversion officer makes no notations about the level of Harris' depression (major, minor or minimal) and, although noting the change of medications, never mentions in the file what is the new antidepressant Harris was prescribed after the Zoloft had been discontinued. Why?

If Harris had smoked marijuana, snorted cocaine or taken any other illegal drug, there seems little doubt that the information would have made it into the file, as in each of the shooter's files the counselors mention having no concerns about illegal drug use. Of course, the shooting at Columbine occurred six years ago, long before the FDA finally acted to place "black box" warnings on antidepressants for adolescent use. But, for the purpose of considering all the pieces to the puzzle—to get an idea about Harris' state of mind—what are the known adverse reactions to mind-altering, psychiatric drugs Zoloft and Luvox?

According to the *PDR*, Zoloft, made by Pfizer Pharmaceuticals, is a selective serotonin reuptake inhibitor (SSRI) and is "presumed" to do something with the chemicals in the brain and "the efficacy of Zoloft in pediatric patients ages 6-17 with major depressive disorder, panic disorder, PTSD (Post Traumatic Stress Disorder), PMDD (Premenstrual Dysphoric Disorder) or social anxiety disorder *has not been established*."[13] (italics mine)

Given that Zoloft has *not* been proven effective in the treatment of major depressive disorder in adolescents, which presumably is the alleged mental disorder for which Harris was diagnosed (depression), investigators might consider this important. But what are the known adverse reactions to the mind-altering drug? Pfizer admits that "during pre-marketing testing, hypomania or mania occurred in approximately 0.4% of the Zoloft treated patients."[14] Mania is defined as "violent abnormal behavior," and hypomania is a milder state of mania.

Because Zoloft has not been approved for use in adolescents with major depressive disorder, Pfizer does not list the dosage information for adolescents with the alleged mental disorder. However, Zoloft is approved for adolescent use for obsessive compulsive disorder

(OCD) and the recommended dose is as follows; "treatment should be initiated with a dose of 25mg once daily in children (6-12) and at a dose of 50mg once daily in adolescents (7-17)." No mention is made in Harris' file about the dosage of Zoloft, but apparently, the mind-altering drug was not working and Harris' mental-health professional decided to switch to another SSRI antidepressant, Luvox.

Luvox, the second mind-altering drug Harris was prescribed, is manufactured by Solvay Pharmaceuticals Inc., and although today is available in countries around the world, the drug was pulled from the U.S. market in 2002 because of "FDA Exclusivity Expiration." Luvox is another of the SSRI class of psychiatric mind-altering drugs and, according to the pharmaceutical company's labeling; among the adverse reactions in pediatric patients "hypomania and mania" are listed. Other noted adverse reactions to Luvox include: *amnesia, manic reaction, psychotic reaction, depression, delirium, delusion, depersonalization, euphoria, hallucinations, hostility, paranoid reaction, phobia, psychosis, sleep disorder, and obsessions.*

While few would argue that Harris' actions were those of someone experiencing some kind of psychotic episode, is it also possible that Harris could have been suffering from a drug-induced psychosis—a manic reaction to the mind-altering drug Luvox, perhaps? Investigators make no mention of this important element of the case, despite the fact that the assault was planned during the time that Harris had been prescribed two mind-altering psychiatric drugs that had *not* been approved for adolescent use in the treatment of depression.

Certainly there are mental-health experts who will argue that Harris' partner, Klebold, had not been diagnosed with an alleged mental disorder and had not been under the influence of mind-altering drugs but still participated in the massacre. This is a valid argument, but some might also argue this is further proof of the illegitimacy of psychiatric diagnosing. But the point, of course, is to examine *all* the information that may assist investigators in understanding the reasons behind the senseless killings.

For example, if the two shooters had dropped acid or taken any other illegal mind-altering drugs prior to the assault, it seems certain that investigators would have made that information part of the investigative discussions. Illegal mind-altering drugs may elicit the same or similar adverse reactions as many of the newer mind-altering antidepressants, yet this important correlation, beyond a cursory mention, is absent from serious consideration in most of the school shootings.

The following list of school shootings is an example of the number of children with a known history of psychiatric counseling and psychiatric drug use. Those "shooters" whose psychiatric background and psychiatric drug use is "unknown" does not mean there is no psychiatric history or psychiatric drug use but, rather, that the public has not been given this information. Despite numerous reports of psychiatric drug use among the "unknown" category, and after unsuccessful attempts to contact attorneys, public defenders and even family members, the psychiatric drug use is only included if it can be directly sourced.

- **Barry Loukaitas**, 14 years old, Feb 2, 1996, Frontier Junior High School, Moses Lake, Wash. Killed a teacher and two students, and wounded another student. Psychiatric drug use: Unknown.

- **Evan Ramsey**, 16 years old, Feb 19, 1997, Bethel High School, Bethel, Pa. Killed one student and one teacher; wounded 2 others. Psychiatric drug use: Unknown.

- **Luke Woodham**, 16 years old, Oct 1, 1997, Pearl High School, Pearl Miss. Killed his mother and two students; wounded seven others. Psychiatric drug use: Unknown.

- **Michael Carneal,** 14 years old, Dec 1, 1997, Heath High School, West Paducah, Ky. Killed three students; wounded five others. Had psychiatric counseling prior to shooting. Psychiatric drug use: Unknown.

- **Mitchell Johnson,** 13 years old, and **Andrew Golden,** 11 years old, March 25, 1998, Westside Middle School, Jonesboro, Ark. One teacher, four students killed; 11 wounded. Psychiatric drug Use: Unknown. Johnson received psychiatric treatment prior to the shooting, and when asked about psychiatric drug use Johnson's attorney, Val Price, said "I think that is confidential information, and I don't want to reveal that."

- **Andrew Wurst**, 14 years old, April 24, 1998, J.W. Parker Middle School, Edinboro, Pa. Killed one teacher; wounded three others. Psychiatric drug use: Unknown.

- **Kipland "Kip" Kinkle,** 15 years old, May 21, 1998, Thurston Middle School, Springfield, Ore. Killed his mother and father and two students; wounded 25 others. Psychiatric counseling and drug use: Prozac.

* **Shawn Cooper**, 15 years old, April 16, 1999, Notus Junior-Senior High School, Notus, Idaho. Fired two gun shots. No one injured or killed. Psychiatric drugs used: "antidepressants."

- **Eric Harris and Dylan Klebold,** 18 and 17 years old, respectively, April 20, 1999, Columbine High School, Littleton, Colo. Twelve students and one teacher killed; 24 others wounded. Shooters commit suicide. Psychiatric drug use: Harris had been prescribed Zoloft and Luvox.

- **Thomas "T.J." Solomon,** 15 years old, May 20, 1999, Heritage High School, Conyers, Ga. Six wounded. Psychiatric drug use: Prior psychiatric counseling and Ritalin.

- **Charles "Andy" Williams,** 15 years old, March 5, 2001, Santana High School, Santee, Calif. Two dead; 13 wounded. Psychiatric drug use: No psychiatric history or psychiatric drug use (Public Defender's office).

- **Elizabeth Bush,** 14 years old, March 7, 2001, Bishop Neumann High School, Williamsport, Pa. Wounded one student. Psychiatric drug use: "antidepressants."

- **Jason Hoffman,** 18 years old, March 22, 2001, Granite Hills High School, El Cajon, Ca. Killed one; wounded one. Psychiatric drug use: Celexa and Effexor.

- **Cory Baadsgaard,** 16 years old, April 15, 2001, Wahluke High School, Mattawa, Wash. Held 23 students and a teacher hostage with a rifle. No injuries or deaths. Psychiatric drug use: Paxil and Effexor.

- **John Jason McLaughlin,** 15-years old, September 14, 2001, Recori High School, Cold Spring, Minnesota. One killed and 1 wounded. Psychiatric drug use: Unknown.

- **Jeff Weise,** 16 years old, March 21, 2005, Red Lake High School, Red Indian Reservation, Minn. Killed nine and wounded seven others then committed suicide. Psychiatric drug use: Prozac.

- **Ken Bartley Jr.,** 15 years old, Nove. 8, 2005, Campbell County High School, Knoxville, Tenn. One principal killed, two assistant principals wounded. Psychiatric drug use: Unknown. Had been placed in a residential counseling program at age 12.

Of these 17 school shootings, eight of the shooters had a known history of psychiatric mind-altering drug use. Three others—Mitchell Johnson, Ken Bartley Jr. and Michael Carneal—had known histories of psychiatric counseling, which more often than not includes psychiatric drug use. Only one shooter, Charles "Andy" Williams, has been confirmed as having had no psychiatric counseling or psychiatric drug history. What about the others? Despite the fact that nearly half of the recent school shooters were using prescribed psychiatric mind-altering drugs; officials continue to refuse to ask the question. But it goes even deeper. Repeated attempts to obtain the information from family members and attorneys were ignored.

Although one can understand why a parent whose child had killed would not welcome such inquiries, on the other hand, those parents might also consider it valuable information to pass along in the hope of finding answers to the horrific assaults. Worse yet, the top bananas in law enforcement, education and mental health have conducted extensive investigations into the school shooting phenomena and the single item conspicuously missing from these reports is the use of psychiatric drugs.

For example, in October 2000 the U.S. Secret Service, in collaboration with the U.S. Department of Education, released a report titled *"An Interim Report on the Prevention of Targeted Violence in Schools,"* which was an intensive investigation into school shootings with the intent of providing some understanding of the attacks and hopefully preventing future events. The 60-page Interim Report discusses many aspects of the shooters' lives but, despite having such detailed information as the shooters' health records, failed to make mention of psychiatric drug use.

Interestingly enough, after I wrote an article about the Interim Report in the May 21, 2001, edition of *Insight on the News* magazine acknowledging that the federal agency failed to mention the possibility of psychiatric drug use by the shooters, in May 2002, nearly two years after the release of the Interim Report, a "Final Report" was released, which was identical to the Interim Report except for a new section about the shooters' mental health status.

The Secret Service's Final Report does not provide specific information such as which shooter was receiving psychiatric counseling or taking psychiatric drugs. Rather, the Final Report explains "The only information collected that would indicate whether attackers had been prescribed psychiatric medications concerned medication noncompliance (i.e., failure to take medication as prescribed). Ten percent of the attackers were known to be noncompliant with prescribed psychiatric medications."[15] The Secret Service does not provide the public with the identities of the individuals who make up the "10 percent" who were "noncompliant."

Not to be outdone by the Secret Service, the FBI conducted its own investigation into school shooters, releasing its September 2000 report titled, *"The School Shooter: A Threat Assessment Perspective."* The FBI, utilizing some of the best and brightest in law enforcement, education and mental health, also failed to raise the issue of psychiatric drug use among the school shooters. Unlike the Secret Service, though, the FBI apparently did not feel compelled to update its report, and it remains today void of any discussion about the shooters' mental health history and psychiatric drug use.

This apparent lack of interest in the use of mind-altering drugs by adolescent shooters seems odd. After all, it isn't as if it is just one or two of the shooters were taking psychiatric drugs. No. Nearly half of the last 17 school shootings involved adolescents who were known to be taking at least one psychiatric drug, and some more than one. This is troubling on a most basic level. Consider for a moment the possibility that nearly half of the school shooters had snorted cocaine prior to their murderous assaults. Does anyone believe that law enforcement would not focus on the illegal drug use? Of course this would be important information to at least note and, in fact, might be considered irresponsible had it not been included. Yet, despite the well-known adverse reactions to the now commonly prescribed psychiatric mind-altering drugs, law enforcement has apparently gone deaf, dumb and blind to this element.

While the adverse reactions to these drugs have been known since the drugs first were approved by the FDA, an argument could be made that no attention has been paid to the dangerous, even potentially life-threatening, adverse effects of the psychiatric drugs because no official stand had been taken on them. With the FDA's recent "black box" warning (Chapter 1), this no longer is true and one might expect the question to be at the top of the list for any investigator looking into a school shooting. Yet, the most recent attack—that of Ken Bartley Jr. in Knoxville, Tenn., on Nov. 8, 2005—continues down the path of all the previous school shootings; whether 15-year-old Bartley was on psychiatric drugs remains a mystery.

There are many questions beyond whether or not a school shooter had been prescribed a psychiatric mind-altering drug that remain unanswered—the least of which is: Does the public have a right to know which students daily are taking dangerous, even life-threatening psychiatric drugs? During a 2001 interview with San Diego Deputy Public Defender William Trainor, whose client was 18-year-old school shooter Jason Hoffman, the boy's then-legal counsel could not say whether the psychiatric drugs (Celexa and Effexor) would be part of his client's defense, but did note "the drugs [Hoffman] was prescribed may help explain his actions."[16]

In the same article, the public defender further added that, "Research indicates that the drugs that were prescribed are extremely powerful antidepressants with the most dangerous side effects." The public defender's remarks were a light at the end of a very dark tunnel: Not only did he "get it" about the dangers of the drugs, but he also understood the implications for those who follow this line of defense. "If you say those drugs may be involved," said Trainor, "you'll be labeled a kook. But with the history of these drugs there is a huge unpredictability factor. When someone goes off while on these drugs it should raise some eyebrows in the community. I'm starting to wonder when the public has the right to this information. What is the balance of rights? It's his [Hoffman] medical records verses the public right to be safe. Which one has the trump card? It is a legitimate question."[17]

It's more than a legitimate question. In fact, it's brilliant and someone needs to make this guy the freaking director of the FBI! Not only did this obscure public servant consider *all* of the information and suggest the possibility of a correlation between the psychiatric drugs and the violent act, he even took a walk on the wild side and asked the question that inexplicably has been missed by the deep thinkers in Washington: Does the public have a right to know which children are taking psychiatric mind-altering drugs? Is psychiatric drug use a public safety issue?

Put another way, one has to wonder what the public's reaction would be to that question if it knew that 16 of the last 17 school shootings involved kids who were taking prescribed mind-altering psychiatric drugs known to cause violent and aggressive behaviors in an unknown percentage of the adolescent population. Of course, this question will remain unanswered until the public demands *all* the information about the school shooters. But defense attorneys never had to make the decision about using the psychiatric drug information in the defense of Jason Hoffman, nor debate the all important question. Ten months after pleading guilty to the charges, Hoffman committed suicide in his jail cell.

But a startling turn of events by our good neighbors across the sea may be, by default, the nail in the coffin that ends the need for debate. In September 2005, the U.K.'s National Health Service along with the National Institute for Clinical Excellence (NICE) formulated guidelines that in effect told British physicians to stop prescribing mind-altering antidepressants to children younger than 18 and recommended exercise and diet as treatment in mild and moderate cases of depression.

Tim Kendall, joint director of the National Collaborating Centre for Mental Health, who led the formulation of the new guidelines, was quoted in a interview with *The Guardian* newspaper as saying "no child, however severe the depression, should have their first line treatment with a drug." Kendall added, "But then if there is any significant risk, we should be offering individual cognitive behavior therapy, depending on their needs. We're really serious that we don't think these drugs should be used lightly."[18] In effect, the Europeans have made it clear that prescribing children mind-altering antidepressants could be harmful and is no longer acceptable as the first line of treatment.

Meanwhile, as the British take decisive steps to curtail the use of the potentially life-threatening drugs, back at the FDA ranch the psycho-pharma cowboys are kicking up their spurs because it only took them a decade to "request" that the pharmaceutical companies place "black box" warnings on the mind-altering drugs. Given that the European community has said "No" to the psychiatric drugging of its children, one might rightly conclude that its high noon for the federal drug slingers in the U.S. and, until they trade the black for the white hat, bloody killing sprees reminiscent of the Wild West are bound to be repeated on high school campuses across the country. Recent history has shown it is not a matter of if, but rather when, another school shooting will occur.

But in the wake of the revelation that Jeff Weise had been on Prozac when he went on his shooting spree at the Red Lake Indian Reservation, maybe it is appropriate to ponder the life-changing event of one boy who narrowly escaped becoming another adolescent with innocent blood on his hands. In April 2001, 16-year-old Cory Baadsgaard took a rifle to Wahluke High School in Washington state and held 23 classmates and a teacher hostage. While Baadsgaard gripped the rifle, classmates calmly talked to him and school intervention specialists were able to enter the room and coax the would-be shooter into putting down the gun.

The 16-year-old does not remember taking the weapon to school and holding his English honors class hostage, and the possible deadly incident is a complete blank to Baadsgaard. The incident occurred just 21 days after the 16-year-old, having been diagnosed as depressed, had been cold-turkeyed off the antidepressant Paxil and had been switched to extraordinarily high doses (300 milligrams) of another mind-altering, psychiatric drug, Effexor.

Paxil, an SSRI manufactured by GlaxoSmithKline, has *not* been approved by the FDA for adolescents diagnosed with a depressive disorder, and according to the *PDR*, some of the known adverse reactions to the drug include; *abnormal thinking, hallucinations, hostility, lack of emotion, manic reaction, neurosis, paranoid reaction, antisocial reaction, delirium, delusions, hysteria, manic-depressive reactions, psychotic depression and psychosis.*

In June 2003 the U.K.'s Department of Health issued a press release informing doctors that Paxil (Seroxat in the U.K.) is not to be prescribed to children under the age of 18 for depressive disorders because the health agency found an increase in the rate of self-harm and potentially suicidal behavior in this group.

The FDA followed up with a June 19, 2003, "Talk Paper" which stated, "There is currently no evidence that Paxil is effective in children or adolescents with MDD (Major Depressive Disorder), and Paxil is not currently approved for use in children and adolescents." The FDA further states "three well-controlled trials in pediatric patients with MDD failed to show that the drug was more effective than placebo (sugar pill)." [19]

The other mind-altering drug 16-year-old Baadsgaard had been prescribed is Effexor, both an SSRI and SNRI (selective norepinephrine reuptake inhibitor) manufactured by Wyeth Pharmaceuticals Inc., which the *PDR* lists the following known adverse reactions; *insomnia, nervousness, anxiety, abnormal dreams, euphoria, hallucinations, hostility, manic reaction, psychosis, delusions, dementia, paranoid reaction, psychotic depression, and suicidal ideation.*

Wyeth Pharmaceuticals' most recent Effexor package insert lists the same frightening adverse reactions and now includes another, "*homicidal ideation,*" which could help explain Baadsgaard's bizarre, out-of-character actions. What is interesting to note from the *PDR* is that Wyeth Pharmaceuticals has this to say about treatment dosages: "In out-patient settings there was no evidence of usefulness of doses greater than 225 mg/day for moderately depressed patients." The pharmaceutical company limits doses to 375 milligrams per day and, yet, 16-year-old Baadsgaard was taking 300 milligrams per day—nearly the maximum allowable limit for adults suffering from depression.

In June 2003, the United Kingdom effectively banned the use of Effexor (venlafaxine HCl) in children after a study found that the drug could cause hostility, suicidal ideas and self-harm. According to a "Dear Health Care Professional" letter distributed by Wyeth to U.K. physicians, "safety and effectiveness in pediatric patients (individuals below 18 years of age) have not been established. In pediatric trials, there were increased reports of hostility and, especially in Major Depressive Disorder, suicide-related adverse events such as suicidal ideation and self-harm." Effexor has *not* been approved by the FDA for use by adolescents suffering from depressive disorders.

Given the above known adverse reactions to the two antidepressant psychiatric drugs, does it seem possible that the drugs could have played a major role in Baadsgaard's actions? In October 2002, I interviewed Baadsgaard's father, Jay, for an *Insight* magazine article titled *"Prescription Drugs May Trigger Killing."* The 16-year-old's father has little doubt about what had driven his son to violence. "The morning that Cory went to school," explained Jay Baadsgaard, "and did what he did, my wife and I just knew that it had to be something with the drugs. That morning he had taken about 300 milligrams of Effexor, and I thought it was something about him going off one of the drugs and then the high dose of the other. One of Cory's friends told us that Cory was yelling and then he just stopped, looked down and saw the gun in his hand and woke up."

"There is no doubt," says Baadsgaard, "that Cory is lucky not to have gone further and I guess I could blame myself for having the gun available, but if I'd known then just what these drugs could do it would have been the drugs that would not have been in our home. They always talk about how the kids who do these things are the ones who get picked on by the jocks and stuff, but Cory was a jock. He was on the varsity basketball team, played football and golf, and was very popular in school. I pray every night that the media will get a hold of this issue. If Cory had been on PCP the media would say 'Oh, he needs drug rehabilitation,' but because these were prescribed medications they say, 'Oh, it can't be that,' but now we know it can be."

One might say that Baadsgaard is the success story of school shooters. He spent 14 months in jail and, in an ironic twist, it was due to the expert testimony of a psychiatrist about the adverse reactions to the drugs he was taking, that the teenager escaped extended incarceration and was released from jail under community supervision for five years. Along with his traumatized classmates, Baadsgaard survived to tell the story. How many others won't?

[1] Monica Davey and Gardiner Harris, "Family Wonders if Prozac Prompted School Shootings" *New York Times*, March 26, 2005.

[2] Physicians' Desk Reference, PDR 2005 59 Edition, Eli Lilly Prozac, pp.1873-78.

[3] Ibid, pp. 1873-78

[4] Ibid, pp. 1873-78

[5] U.S. Food and Drug Administration, "FDA Alert 07/2005 –Suicidal Thoughts or Actions in Children and Adults.

[6] Wikipedia Internet Enclyclopedia: Eric Harris and Dylan Klebold.

[7] Robert Kriegshauser, Termination Report Juvenile Diversion 2/3/99 Dylan Klebold.

[8] Jefferson County Juvenile Diversion Program File, 2/3/99 Dylan Klebold.

[9] Termination Report Juvenile Diversion 3/25/99 Eric Harris

[10] Ibid.

[11] Ibid.

[12] Ibid.

[13] Physicians' Desk Reference 2005 Edition 59, Pfizer, Zoloft, pp.2684.

[14] Ibid, pp. 2683

[15] The Final Report and Findings of the Safe School Initiative: Implications for the Prevention of School Attacks in the United States., U.S. Secret Service, U.S. Department of Education. May 2002.

[16] Kelly Patricia O'Meara, "A Prescription for Violence?" *Insight* Magazine, May 21, 2001.

[17] Ibid.

[18] Sarah Boseley, Health Editor, *Guardian*, September 28, 2005.

[19] Food and Drug Administration, FDA Talk Paper "FDA Statement Regarding the Anti-Depressant Paxil for Pediatric Population." June, 19, 2003.

Chapter Six

A Drug by Any Other Name

There are a few things in life that most people can agree on, including the very basic desire to feel good, whether it be physically or mentally. The problem, though, is that life is full of ups and downs, and bad things happen to good people. As the Rolling Stones lyrics so aptly explain, "You can't always get what you want."

Put simply, save for an extraordinarily lucky few, for a host of reasons sometimes life really sucks. The question that remains is how to deal with the mental/emotional highs and lows that can affect the quality of life just as seriously as any medical condition. While the psycho-wizards would have us believe that being depressed, or any other psychiatric diagnosis, is a disease of the brain, in reality there is no medical or scientific proof to support this conclusion—no disease, an objective, confirmable abnormality.

Nevertheless, the psycho-pharmaceutical industrial complex, through clever—and what some might call deceptive—advertising campaigns, has successfully convinced an ever-increasing number of Americans that their mental/emotional troubles *are* abnormalities of the brain, such as the well-known yet theoretical chemical imbalance. Moreover, psychiatric mind-altering drugs have been created and sold as "treatments" for these alleged mental abnormalities but, in reality, the pharmaceutical companies admit they do not understand how the drugs "work" for the alleged abnormality and, worse still, the drugs actually disrupt the naturally occurring chemicals in the brain. Still Americans are led to believe they'll be "better" if they take the "treatment." Never-ending happiness in a pill? Wow! It sounds good. But is it that simple, or is it too good to be true?

Up to this point the majority of information about the fraud of psychiatric diagnosing and the dangers associated with psychiatric mind-altering drugs primarily has focused on adolescent use, the adverse effects of the drugs and how these potentially life-threatening effects may or may not play a role in violent, suicidal/ homicidal behavior. Recall that in 2004 the FDA warned the public that there was an "increased risk of suicidal thoughts and behavior" in adolescents who take psychiatric mind-altering drugs, and the federal drug approval agency even went so far as to officially alert the public stating that "children taking antidepressants may increase suicidal thoughts and actions in about 1 out of 50 people 18 years or younger."

This is a sobering figure, given that millions of children are taking antidepressants, suggesting that the number of ticking time bombs among us should cause serious concern and, at a minimum, raise questions about the approval process of drugs that are potentially life-threatening to an unknown percentage of the population. But the FDA crescendo is its stand on psychiatric mind-altering drugs and adolescent use. The drug approval agency concluded that, after careful consideration of pharmaceutical-company-supplied clinical trial data, the majority of clinical trials the agency reviewed revealed that the psychiatric mind-altering drugs are no more effective than a placebo (sugar pill) in treating the alleged stated mental disorder. An unknown number of the adolescent population is being prescribed mind-altering drugs that are neither safe nor effective.

Okay, let's recap. Neither the APA, the NIMH nor any other scientific/medical organization is capable of providing objective, confirmable data to support the claims that psychiatric diagnoses are abnormalities of the brain. The pharmaceutical companies openly admit they do not understand how the drugs work in the brain for the alleged brain abnormality, and the FDA has warned the public that an unknown percentage of the adolescent population taking these mind-altering drugs may experience self-harm and other violent behaviors.

Doesn't sound too good for American kids, but what about the tens of millions of American adults using these same psychiatric mind-altering drugs for the same alleged mental disorders? Has the adult population been provided *all* the information it needs to make an informed decision about psychiatric drug use? Are psychiatric mind-altering drugs safe and effective for adults?

In the summer of 2005, a mere eight months after the FDA warned the public about the possible dangers associated with mind-altering psychiatric drugs for adolescents, the deep thinkers at the drug approval agency charged with ensuring that the approved drugs are safe *and* effective, felt compelled to release another "Public Health Advisory" warning of "an increased risk for suicidal behavior in adults who are being treated with antidepressant medications."[1] Specifically, the FDA highlighted that:

- Adults being treated with antidepressant medications, particularly those being treated for depression, should be watched closely for worsening of depression and for increased suicidal thinking or behavior. Close watching may be especially important early in treatment, or when the dose is changed, either increased or decreased.

- Adults whose symptoms worsen while being treated with antidepressant drugs, including an increase in suicidal thinking or behavior, should be evaluated by their health care professional.

This is interesting information on a number of levels, the least of which involves the realization that an extraordinarily large number of Americans are prescribed mind-altering drugs for the alleged mental illness depression, yet the FDA appears to be warning that the psychiatric antidepressant drugs may worsen depression in adults— to the point of becoming suicidal. This warning becomes even more, well, depressing when one considers that potential clinical trial participants for drug studies are excluded early in the screening process if they are, or have been, suicidal—further suggesting that it is the mind-altering drugs that cause the increased suicidal thoughts, not the alleged psychiatric diagnosis of depression.

Peter Breggin, M.D., a court-qualified medical expert who has more than 30 years in private practice in psychiatry, has participated in numerous private liability lawsuits and is the author of dozens of scientific reports and books, including *Talking Back to Prozac* and *Your Drug May Be Your Problem,* understands the tricks of the clinical trial trade and further raises questions about the FDA's commitment to the public's safety.

"The most serious cases of depression," explains Breggin, "almost always are excluded from the clinical trials and, for example, the clinical trials for antidepressants almost always occur as outpatient trials, where they exclude in-patients. They always exclude patients who have a significant suicide risk and those who have a diagnosis of manic depressive disorder. So, the patients who are in these trials represent a lower risk of severe depression and suicidality and other abnormal mental responses than do many patients in routine clinical practice. In addition, the trials are very limited in their ability to pick up adverse reactions because they generally only last four to six weeks. Overall, if you can get a serious, dangerous signal of something like mania, suicidality or violence in a clinical trial you can be almost certain that the risk in actual practice is much more frequent and severe. There is no doubt whatsoever that the SSRIs increase suicidality in adults and, in fact, I have data that I've obtained from looking inside more than one of the manufacturers of these drugs, indicating an increased suicide attempt rate in materials that have not been fully evaluated by the FDA. Initially the material was withheld by the pharmaceuticals then, when made public, the FDA showed no interest in the material."

"More than that," says Breggin, "when I announced during my testimony at the 2004 FDA public hearings that I had this material on increased suicidality from looking at these private records of these companies during private liability suits, I invited the FDA to please talk to me about it. [But] they never got in touch with me. The FDA doesn't want to hear about the mistakes. During the time when anonymous documents showed up in the *British Medical Journal* (Jan. 1, 2005, issue) one of the documents indicated that in the clinical trials for Prozac there was an increased rate of suicidality in patients compared to both the older antidepressants and the placebo used during the clinical trials. Eli Lilly had the data from the beginning, but the FDA did not have the data when they were conducting the 1991 public hearings."

Breggin is referring to confidential clinical trial drug data and physician notes obtained by and published in the *British Medical*

Journal (*BMJ*) in January 2005, which questioned pharmaceutical giant Eli Lilly's safety claims about Prozac (fluoxetine HCl), the mother of all psycho-pharmacological interventions. Among the documents reported by freelance journalist Jeanne Lenzer in the *BMJ* include "a report of 8 November 1988," entitled "Activation and Sedation in Fluoxetine Clinical Trials," that found that in clinical trials "38% of fluoxetine-treated patients reported new activation but 19% of placebo-treated patients also reported new activation, yielding a difference of 19% attributable to fluoxetine."[2]

In psycho-pharma-speak, "activation" refers to adverse drug reactions such as agitation, insomnia and extreme inner nervousness which, according to the Lilly documents as reported in the *BMJ*, twice as many clinical trial participants experienced while taking the mind-altering Prozac compared to those receiving the placebo. Immediately following the publication of the *BMJ* article, Eli Lilly demanded and received a correction as well as an apology from the *BMJ* for the portion of the article which referred to the suggestion that the mentioned confidential documents had gone "missing," not disputing whether the information contained in the documents was factually correct.

In fact, Eli Lilly placed costly full-page advertisements in the nation's leading newspapers to respond to the *BMJ* article, but nowhere in Lilly's ad does the pharmaceutical giant state that the information contained in the "missing" documents is factually incorrect. The point of contention then appears to be when the seemingly damning information was available for FDA review and public consumption. According to an Associated Press report, *BMJ* Editor Kamran Abbasi said, "whether or not Eli Lilly made all of the information available to the FDA at the appropriate times is a question for the FDA to answer...[W]e await their response."[3]

Just when the "missing" documents were provided to the U.S. drug approval agency has yet to be determined and, at the time of this writing, it has been nearly a full year since the FDA took this matter under consideration, conducting a review of just when the aforementioned documents were provided by Eli Lilly. Naturally, there is a great deal at stake. Consider for a moment the possible outcomes. First, Eli Lilly very well could have provided the FDA the documentation about the adverse reactions (suicidality) found during the clinical trials, as well as the information passed along to Lilly by German physicians reviewing the drug prior to the U.S. approval of Prozac. But the FDA either overlooked the negative findings or the adverse findings simply were lost in the thousands of pages of information the FDA routinely receives with new drug applications. In either instance, it would appear that the FDA dropped the ball. On the other hand, Eli Lilly quite possibly did not provide the FDA with this important data when applying for drug approval or the data were presented in such a scattered manner that its significance was lost on the FDA reviewer.

Whether Colonel Mustard did it in the library with the lead pipe still is a mystery. One might expect the well-funded FDA to have at its disposal an efficient "we-can-find-anything" filing system, but still the agency has not completed its review of the matter. Really, how difficult can this be? Prozac was approved by the FDA in December 1987. It would make sense that the FDA would be troubled with reviewing only the documentation provided by Eli Lilly *prior* to December 1987, you know, just the documents that are part of the Prozac approval file. After all, any documentation received after that date would suggest that Prozac was approved without FDA knowledge of the adverse reactions mentioned in the questioned "missing" documents. The FDA did not respond to my inquiries about the status of its review.

Regardless of the fact that Blockbuster Video apparently could provide the FDA lessons on data filing and retrieval, it appears that the outcome of the review very well may fall on the side of the FDA. In response to questions raised about the reported "missing" Eli Lilly documents, Richard Kapit M.D., the doctor who reviewed Prozac data for FDA approval in 1987, told the *BMJ* "if we have good evidence that we were misled and that data was withheld, then I would change my mind. I do agree now that these stimulatory side effects, especially in regard to suicidal and homicidal ideation, are worse than I thought at the time that I reviewed the drug."[4]

"Worse than I thought at the time that I reviewed the drug?" The good doctor did not elaborate on this astonishing statement, but one has to wonder just what information Kapit had at the time of the approval of the sale of Prozac in the U.S. that apparently went from bad to "worse" in the following decade. Nevertheless there are plenty of clues that provide interesting insight into Kapit's remarks, and some of them had been around long before the 1987 approval of Prozac.

The following internal Eli Lilly documents were introduced during the 1999 "Forsyth trial." Bill Forsyth had been on Prozac for just nine days when he stabbed his wife 15 times, killing her and, with the same knife, ending his own life. [5] The Forsyth family believed their father's homicidal/suicidal actions were the result of adverse effects of Prozac. Among information contained in the documents:

- **May 1984:** BGA comments (German Regulatory Authority) – "During the treatment with the preparation [Prozac] 16 suicides were made, 2 of these with success. As patients with a risk of suicide were excluded from the studies, it is probable that this high proportion can be attributed to an action of the preparation [Prozac]..."
- **March 29, 1985:** Benefit/Risk Consideration – "the incidence rate [suicide] under fluoxetine [Prozac] therefore purely mathematically is 5.6 times higher than under the other active medication imipramine... The benefits vs. risks considerations for fluoxetine [Prozac] currently do not fall clearly in favor of the benefits. Therefore it is of the greatest importance that it be determined whether there is a particular subgroup of patients who respond better to fluoxetine [Prozac] than to imipramine, so that the higher incidence of suicide attempts may be tolerable."
- **June 1986:** Draft of proposed "Precaution and Adverse Reactions" sections of the Prozac package insert—"Mania and psychosis may be precipitated in susceptible patients by antidepressant therapy." (Never included in actual inserts.)

- **August 1989:** Additional feedback regarding the fluoxetine [Prozac] review by the Commission A [Germany] The counterindication because of acute suicidality should become a warning whereby the physicians should be advised that in the absence of sedation, the risk of higher suicidality should be taken into account."

- **August 3, 1990:** Letter to sales representatives regarding reports of suicidal ideation/behavior possibly associated with Prozac therapy—"This information is not intended to replace our current promotional strategy but is being provided to enable you to respond to physicians when appropriate. You should not initiate discussion on these issues nor use this letter in detailing. However, if asked to comment on these issues by a health-care professional, you should: 1. Reassure the healthcare professional that no casual relationship has been established between suicidal ideation and Prozac therapy."

- **October 2, 1990:** Memo of Lilly employee Leigh Thompson to Lilly employee Robert Zerbe regarding an upcoming Prozac symposium in which the issue of suicidality is discussed: "Then the question is what to do with the "big" numbers on suicidality. If the report numbers are shown next to those for nausea, they seem small."

- **November 13, 1990:** Memo from Claude Bouchy (Lilly Germany) to Leigh Thompson Re: Adverse Drug Event Reporting: Suicide Fluoxetine – In response to Lilly's request that he [Bouchy] change the event "suicidal ideation" to "depression," Bouchy writes: "Hans, [another Lilly employee in Germany] has medical problems with these directions and I have great concerns about it. I do not think I could explain to a BGA, a judge, to a reporter or even to my family why we would do this, especially on the sensitive issue of suicide and suicidal ideation."

- **November 14, 1990:** Second memo from Bouchy to Thompson Re: Adverse Drug Event Reporting – Suicide Fluoxetine, in which he states: "I personally wonder whether we are really helping the credibility of an excellent ADE system by calling [an] overdose what a physician reports as suicide attempt and by calling depression what a physician is reporting as suicide ideation."

- **1995:** Dr. Jick's Study, "Antidepressants and Suicide" – "The results indicate that only fluoxetine [Prozac] has a rate that seems to be substantially higher than that of the other antidepressants."

Based on these Eli Lilly internal documents it appears that the company had a clear idea about suicidality and harmful behavior associated with Prozac, and certainly prior to the U.S. approval of the drug. More than that, it also appears that the concern within the company was great enough that pressure was being exerted on drug reviewers to change adverse event language, which many might surmise was an attempt to disguise the negative outcomes being reported by physicians. The question, though, is whether the above internal documents were made available to Prozac reviewer Kapit or anyone at the FDA. This is no small matter when one considers that the FDA does not conduct its own tests on pending drugs but, rather, relies on supposedly complete and honest data provided by the drug companies to make drug approval decisions.

Peter Breggin was the plaintiffs' medical and scientific expert in an earlier 1994 lawsuit brought by victims of Joseph Wesbecker, who killed eight and wounded 12 others before taking his own life. Wesbecker had been on Prozac for just one month when the shooting occurred. In response to the brouhaha over the *BMJ* article, Breggin stepped up to the plate to clarify what he believed to be the facts about the "missing" documents.

In a January 2005 report titled *"An Examination of Eli Lilly and Company's Contentions that the BMJ Prozac Documents were Never Missing and Have No Significance,"* Breggin contradicts the pharmaceutical giant's assertions that the questioned "missing" documents have been made publicly available and, in 12 specific points, reveals the lengths the pharmaceutical giant was willing to go in its quest to get and keep Prozac on the market (in part):

"Eli Lilly never provided these important documents or any equivalent of them to the FDA, to other medical authorities or to professional publications in the interest of public health. Eli Lilly fought to keep them from surfacing, and when forced by litigation to offer them as discovery, the drug company settled cases and sealed the documents in order to avoid the documents becoming public. Until the release of these documents by the BMJ, Eli Lilly succeeded for many years in keeping each of these documents from surfacing. Despite their great public health importance, until now these documents have been largely unknown to the FDA, the legal profession, the medical and scientific community and the public."[6]

According to Breggin's recollection, the FDA most definitely was left out of the Lilly loop during the drug agency's 1987 Prozac approval review. And, although Lilly succeeded in getting FDA approval, recall that just three years later, in 1991, the FDA was forced to hold hearings about the possibility that the new class of antidepressants, selective serotonin reuptake inhibitors, Lilly's Prozac being the first, were causing suicidality and other harmful behaviors. Were these damning internal Lilly documents made available to the 1991 FDA review committee? Breggin's examination still finds the federal drug approval agency "loop less" on the Lilly documents (in part):

"Lilly had completed and possessed all of the documents at the 1991 FDA PDAC hearing, whose purpose was to evaluate the risk of antidepressant-induced suicidality. The only item produced from among all the documents was a single graph about hostility and intentional injury from the FDA's spontaneous reporting system. It was flashed on the screen by the FDA representative, never discussed, and then went missing at the FDA. Breggin tried to obtain that document before and after the Wesbecker case, and was finally told by letter from the FDA that they couldn't find it. In addition, and very important, while the FDA did show the hostility and intentional injury graph at the 1991 PDAC meeting, the agency did not show

the dramatic graphs and tables concerning Prozac-induced suicide attempt, overdose and psychotic depression. Eli Lilly did not produce any information concerning these graphs at the meeting."[7]

So let's recap. According to Dr. Breggin's breakdown of the *BMJ* "missing" documents, the FDA had not been provided important medical information about the potentially deadly adverse effects of Prozac before the drug's approval in 1987, and these same data also were not available for consideration by the FDA during the 1991 review of the SSRIs. Based on the above, many may conclude that Eli Lilly, in the immortal words of Ricky Ricardo, has "some splainen to do!"

Still, though, there is the matter of the 2004 public hearings, where once again, due to the public outcry, the FDA was forced to revisit the issue of suicidality and SSRIs due to an ever-increasing number of claims that the mind-altering antidepressants (including Prozac) were causing suicidal thoughts and other harmful behaviors. What does Breggin conclude?

"Lilly continued to hide the documents and the data at the 2004 FDA hearings on pediatric suicidality caused by antidepressants. At the hearings Tom Laughren of the FDA said that he knew of no data linking SSRIs to suicide or hostility. Breggin openly contradicted Laughren during his presentation at the second hearing and told him that suicide data did exist in regard to Prozac. The FDA continued to act unaware of the existence of any such documents in 2004 and did not ask Breggin any details about them."[8]

Based on the above, it appears that Eli Lilly, putting it charitably, has been less than straightforward and some might even conclude that the pharmaceutical giant has a long history of purposefully withholding adverse data about Prozac, subsequently allowing the company to reap the financial windfall from the best-selling antidepressant, despite possessing information that drug reviewers most likely would consider important in the ongoing debate and also would prove useful to the consuming public.

Then again, it's difficult to take seriously any information that would come from the pharmaceutical giant when today, for example, the company continues to report on its website under "Depression" that "Lilly revolutionized the treatment of this debilitating *disease...*"[9] If the psycho-pharma wizards at Lilly cannot differentiate between what is and is not disease (an objective, confirmable abnormality) then one might also question the level of credibility the company is due when it comes to choking up the truth about the side effects of the treatments it peddles.

Nevertheless, it seems fair to say that Eli Lilly is not alone when it comes to juicy internal communications but, given that Prozac was the first of the new class of SSRIs approved by the FDA, one would expect at the very least some degree of integrity on the part of the company in advising the public of possible life-threatening adverse reactions and an even higher degree of scrutiny on the part of the drug approval agency. More to the point, it would seem logical to assume that everyone involved in the approval process of Prozac was aware that the then-new class of antidepressants are serious psychiatric drugs intended to disrupt the balance of the naturally occurring chemicals in the brain and subsequently alter human behavior.

That there are serious adverse reactions associated with the use of Prozac no longer is in question and, certainly, not to the doctors who early on reported the adverse effects to Eli Lilly. Rather, what remains unanswered by the FDA is when the drug agency learned about the adverse effects—suicidality and self-harm—associated with Prozac. Only the FDA can answer that question, and the federal agency appears to be apprehensive or incapable of providing the answer. But the FDA has other ways of learning about adverse reactions to drugs and, in fact, Prozac has been on the FDA's radar screen since the drug first went on the market by way of its adverse event reporting system (AERS), a recordkeeping system whereby patients and physicians record adverse reactions with the drug approval agency.

For example, Eli Lilly reports that more than 54 million patients worldwide have taken Prozac. This figure is impressive. But consider for a moment that of those 54 million patients, FDA data reveals that by 1994 it had received nearly 30,000 adverse event reports, including more than 1,700 deaths with nearly 1,100 of those attributed to suicides and nearly 1,900 suicide attempts. In total, nearly 10 percent of the total adverse drug events (ADEs) for Prozac were attributed to suicides and suicide attempts.[10]

However, if the U.S. Government Accountability Office (GAO) is correct and only 1 percent to 10 percent of the actual adverse events are reported and "are unlikely to be representative of the much larger number of unreported events," then the numbers of adverse events associated with Prozac should be substantially higher.[11]

But is it really necessary to continue to calculate the ever-increasing number of adverse drug events associated with Prozac or any of the SSRI/SNRI antidepressants? After all, how many adverse reports of suicides and attempted suicides does it take to get the FDA's attention? What is the acceptable risk-benefit ratio?

The drug approval agency has been known to pull a drug for far fewer complaints. For instance, it wasn't too many years ago that the FDA pulled from the market the appetite suppressants Fen-Phen (Fenfluramine and Dexfenfluramine) when it became aware of less than 150 adverse reports associated with heart valve damage.

What's up? The FDA received tens of thousands of adverse event reports for Prozac yet today it remains a top selling psychiatric drug, pulling in tens of billions of dollars during its 18 years on the market. In fact, by 1998, Eli Lilly's Prozac held the dubious distinction of garnering the first place slot at the FDA for receiving the most adverse event reports for any of the more than 3,200 drugs on the market. The same year, the "wonder" drug, Prozac, also took home first place for racking up the most reported "serious" side effects.[12] Despite Prozac's dubious standing with the FDA, the pharmaceutical company continues to preach the safety of the mind-altering drug.

Following the *BMJ* "missing" document debacle, the company put out a press release pooh-poohing the very idea that Eli Lilly would withhold any data that would be important to the public's safety: "It has always been Lilly's objective to publicly disclose data about both the safety and efficacy of fluoxetine," and "Lilly is committed to the health and safety of all patients being treated with our medicines and to ensuring healthcare professionals and families have the information they need to make informed treatment decisions."[13]

The pharmaceutical company may be "committed," and full disclosure may be its "objective," but based on the following information, the company's pronouncements fall short on follow-through and raise questions about its commitment to "ensuring healthcare professionals and families have the information they need..." For example, Eli Lilly's exclusive patent rights on fluoxetine (Prozac) expired in August 2001, which would not bode well for the company's revenues. But Lilly had no intention of letting go of the Prozac cash cow: One year prior to Prozac's patent expiration, the FDA approved Lilly's "new" treatment, Sarafem, for premenstrual dysphoric disorder (PMDD).

But what exactly is PMDD? Well, as is the case with all the psychiatric diagnoses, no one really knows, not even Eli Lilly: "While it is unknown what causes PMDD, many doctors believe it may be related to an imbalance in a natural chemical in the body called serotonin." (There it is again, the theoretical chemical imbalance!) As has been well demonstrated throughout this book, there is no known method available for measuring the levels of chemicals or even what are correct levels of serotonin (or any of the naturally occurring chemicals) in the individual human brain. Of course, Lilly is well aware of this fact and, therefore, added the very special caveat "doctors believe."

The fact is this new alleged mental disorder, PMDD, affects only women, and then only a few days out of the month. That's right, this mental illness, exclusively targeting women, comes and goes every two weeks or so. According to the deep thinkers at the APA, the once-monthly female mental illness has not yet become a full-fledged mental disorder in the *Diagnostic and Statistical Manual of Mental Disorders* (*DSM-IV*) but, rather, remains in the manual's appendix as a disorder needing further research. Nevertheless, the *DSM-IV* provides the following symptom criteria for the unofficial PMDD:

- Markedly depressed mood
- Marked anxiety
- Marked affectivity
- Decreased interest in activities
- Feeling tense, anxious or "on edge"

- Persistent irritability, anger and increased inter-personal conflicts
- Feeling fatigued, lethargic or lacking energy
- Marked changes in appetite
- A subjective feeling of being overwhelmed or out of control
- Physical symptoms such as breast tenderness, swelling or bloating

The *DSM-IV* explains that women must experience five or more of the "symptoms" before a psychiatric diagnosis can be made. Lilly's advertising for the then-new "treatment" for PMDD states "doctors can treat PMDD with Sarafem – the first and only prescription medication for PMDD." One might wonder just how an antidepressant can reduce the physical symptoms of breast tenderness, swelling or bloating – does the patient think the symptoms away? It's hard to know because Lilly did not market Sarafem as an antidepressant.

But Sarafem is the antidepressant Prozac under a new name. No more, no less. The only difference between Lilly's mind-altering Prozac and its mind-altering Sarafem is the color of the pill. Lilly apparently at least thought it appropriate to change the color of Prozac from green to the very feminine pink and lavender. The chemical name of Prozac's active ingredient is *fluoxetine HCl*, and the active ingredient in Sarafem is *fluoxetine HCl*.

During an interview in April 2001, I asked a representative of Eli Lilly to explain the difference between Sarafem and Prozac. Laura Miller, a marketing associate for Lilly, explained that the difference in the treatments is in "how women react to the drug." Huh? In an attempt to clarify, Miller explained, "We asked women and physicians about the treatment of PMDD, and they told us they wanted a treatment option with its own identity that would differentiate PMDD from depression. As you know, Prozac is one of the best-known trademarks in the pharmaceutical industry and is closely associated with depression. They wanted a treatment option with its own identity."

This answer, it seemed, insinuated that women didn't mind taking an antidepressant for the once-a-month discomfort; they just didn't want anyone to know it was an antidepressant. Nevertheless, still searching for an answer that specifically addressed my question, I pressed on. "What is the difference if a woman takes 20 milligrams (mg) of Prozac (fluoxetine HCl) for depression or 20 mg of Sarafem (fluoxetine HCl) for PMDD?" Miller then explained, "The difference is that PMDD is a distinct clinical condition different than depression. PMDD is not depression." On this point, Lilly's Miller is mistaken and might want to chat with her psycho-wizard colleagues at the APA, as anyone clearly can see that depression tops the list of "symptoms" for diagnosing the alleged PMDD.

Given that I considered the Lilly spokesperson's answers grossly deficient, evasive and nearly insulting, I tried a more direct approach: "What is the difference if it's the same drug?" Rather than clarify, the Lilly mouthpiece continued on the disorder path, "PMDD is cyclical—women suffer from PMDD up to two weeks before their menses, and the other two weeks of the month they don't have the symptoms of PMDD." There's a new concept, a mental disorder that comes and goes every two weeks or so!

Yes, the answers were a real head-shaker, and I could come to no other conclusion than Miller was doing a good job of Lilly-speak. Talk about making someone crazy, I felt an overwhelming desire to scream, begging her to just say it... SARAFEM IS PROZAC! But it would have done no good. This well-paid servant of the pharmaceutical giant was going to stay on point no matter how silly and personally degrading the answers were.

But it is precisely Miller's answers to straightforward questions that appear to run contradictory to Lilly's "objective" and its "commitment" to "the health and safety of all patients being treated with our medicines and to ensuring healthcare professionals and families have the information they need to make informed treatment decisions." Just how informed are professionals and families if Lilly fails to make crystal clear in its marketing that the drug it is hawking as new—Sarafem—is nothing more than a pink and lavender version of the old green Prozac? But let's be more specific. The labeling information for both Prozac and Sarafem is as follows:

Prozac empirical formula: $C_{17}H_{18}F_3NO \bullet HCl$

$F_3C-\langle\bigcirc\rangle-O-CHCH_2CH_2NHCH_3 \quad \bullet \ HCl$

Sarafem empirical formula: $C_{17}H_{18}F_3NO \bullet HCl$

$F_3C-\langle\bigcirc\rangle-O-CHCH_2CH_2NHCH_3 \quad \bullet \ HCl$

What part of the above formulas is different? Obviously, there is no difference. Even the description of the drug provided by the FDA is identical:

Prozac: "the antidepressant, antiobsessive-compulsive and antibulimic actions of fluoxetine *are presumed to be linked to its inhibition of CNS (central nervous system) neuronal uptake of serotonin.*"

Sarafem: "the mechanism of action of fluoxetine in premenstrual dysphoric disorder (PMDD) is unknown, but *is presumed to be linked to its inhibition of CNS (central nervous system) neuronal uptake of serotonin.*"

It appears that in the world of psychiatric mind-altering drugs, one-size-fits-all is the rule of thumb. In other words, if one suffers from any of the alleged psychiatric diagnoses, including obsessive-compulsive disorder, bulimia, depression or PMDD, fluoxetine HCl (Prozac/Sarafem) is the "treatment." In fact, given that there is no chemical difference between Prozac and Sarafem, a patient seemingly could take Sarafem for depression, bulimia or obsessive-compulsive disorder. After all, the FDA lists both Prozac and Sarafem as antidepressants because both disrupt the naturally occurring chemicals in the brain (the central nervous system) and are subject to the same adverse reactions (suicidal thinking and behavior) contained in the "black box" warnings now listed on all antidepressants.

What is more interesting is that in 2003 Warner Chilcott Pharmaceuticals paid $295 million to acquire the U.S. sales and marketing rights for Sarafem. Listed on the company's Sarafem website (http://www.Sarafem.com) under "Important Safety Information," Warner Chilcott explains: *"Although Sarafem is not a treatment for depression, it contains fluoxetine hydrochloride, the same active ingredient in some antidepressants."* Oh yeah, there's some truth in advertising!

Is Warner Chilcott kidding: "the same active ingredient in *some* antidepressants?" While it is always amusing to see how creative the marketing teams at the pharmaceutical companies can be, let's return for a moment from planet psycho-pharma for a reality check. Is it asking too much to expect the pharmaceutical companies to show the women of America a little respect and just admit that Sarafem is Prozac, the No. 1 selling antidepressant of all time?! It appears that when hundreds of millions of dollars are at stake, the "commitment" and "objective" to be completely open and honest takes a back seat to big bucks.

More than that, how can it possibly be said that Sarafem "is not a treatment for depression?" Sarafem is Prozac, which is marketed and sold as treatment for depression. Whether it actually is effective in "treating" the alleged mental illness of depression is quite another matter. But just for the fun of it, let's consider Warner Chilcott's ridiculous statement for a moment. Suppose a woman is suffering from the alleged psychiatric disorder PMDD and is prescribed Sarafem as treatment, and this same patient also is suffering from depression, wouldn't Sarafem treat the depression? If not, given that the two pills share identical chemical formulas, how then can Prozac be said to treat depression? On the other hand, why not just use Prozac for the alleged PMDD? And, taking it one step further, if a woman is suffering from depression *and* PMDD, does the physician prescribe Prozac for the depression and Sarafem for PMDD – a cocktail of the same drug?

While the above questions may seem silly, they are nevertheless legitimate, especially when one has to wonder just how many treating physicians actually explain to their female patients that the "new" Sarafem is in reality the old Prozac. Of course, if the treating physician did explain to patients that Sarafem actually is Prozac, it would blow the explanation provided by Lilly's mouthpiece that "We asked women and physicians about the treatment of PMDD, and they told us they wanted a treatment option with its own identity."

In order to get a truly amusing glimpse into planet psycho-pharma's theatre of the absurd one only need review Eli Lilly's "Dear Healthcare Professional" letter, **"Prozac – No longer authorized for treatment of Pre-Menstrual Dysphoric Disorder (PMDD),"** which was distributed to all physicians in the United Kingdom in December 2003 (the same month that Lilly sold off its sales and marketing rights of Sarafem to Warner Chilcott). Lilly provided the reason for withdrawing Prozac as treatment for PMDD: "PMDD is not a well-established disease entity across Europe. It is not listed in the International Classification of Diseases (ICD) and remains only a research diagnosis in the American Psychiatric Associations DSM-IV classification..." There it is. Prozac *was* considered a treatment for PMDD in the United Kingdom, at least until 2003. Naturally, anyone with an 8th grade education may be wondering that if Prozac is no longer considered treatment for PMDD, then why is Sarafem considered a "treatment" for PMDD? It is the same drug! More than that, not only is PMDD "not a well-established disease" in the United Kingdom, there is no proof that it is a disease at all—an objective, confirmable, abnormality. So why is Sarafem prescribed to women suffering from the alleged PMDD in the U.S.? PMDD is not "a well-established disease" in the U.S. and, in fact, if it was a brain disease the patient would seek treatment from a neurologist not a psychiatrist.

In the end, regardless of clever, yet, often insulting marketing and unproven mental illnesses, giving a pill a new name and changing its color does not change the fact that Sarafem is the world-famous—and some would say infamous— antidepressant Prozac and subject to the same adverse reactions (suicidality and other harmful behaviors). But pharmaceutical giant Eli Lilly isn't the only pharmaceutical company to switch hit drugs. GlaxoSmithKline also peddle the same drug as treatment for two separate alleged psychiatric diagnoses.

In 1995 the FDA approved for sale GlaxoSmithKline's antidepressant Wellbutrin (bupropion HCl). The drug approval agency's description of the mind-altering drug reads this way (in part): "Bupropion is a relatively weak inhibitor of the neuronal uptake of norepinephrine, serotonin and dopamine…while the mechanism of action of bupropion, as with other antidepressants, *is unknown, it is presumed that this action is mediated by noradrenergic and/or dopaminergic mechanisms."* (italics mine)

Minus all the technical jargon, Wellbutrin is another antidepressant that is "presumed," blah, blah, blah, to do something with the naturally occurring chemicals in the brain. Although Wellbutrin has not been approved for use among children younger than 18 years old, it carries the same "black box" warnings about suicidal thinking and behavior as do all of the other antidepressants available on the market today.

But like Eli Lilly's Prozac/Sarafem, GlaxoSmithKline found a multi-purpose use for its mind-altering Wellbutrin. In 1997, the FDA approved for sale Zyban (bupropion HCl) as a non-nicotine aid to smoking cessation. The FDA approved description of the drug reads this way (in part): "Bupropion is a relatively weak inhibitor of the neuronal uptake of norepinephrine, serotonin, and dopamine… the mechanism by which Zyban enhances the ability of patients to abstain from smoking *is unknown…it is presumed that this action is mediated by noradrenergic and/or dopaminergic mechanisms."* (italics mine)

Save for inserting a different drug name, the alleged mental illness it treats, and of course the routine caveat that nobody knows how the drug works on the alleged mental illness, there is no difference between the description of Wellbutrin and Zyban. The fact is Wellbutrin is Zyban and Zyban is Wellbutrin. More specifically, a cursory examination of the molecular formulas confirms they are the same drug:

Wellbutrin: $C_{13}H_{18}ClNO \bullet HCl$ Zyban: $C_{13}H_{18}ClNO \bullet HCl$

NHC(CH₃)₃

COCHCH₃

• HCl

Cl

NHC(CH₃)₃

COCHCH₃

• HCl

Cl

There is no doubt that Wellbutrin and Zyban are the same drug. And, in fact, the FDA approved prescribing information states in part: "Although Zyban is not indicated for treatment of depression, it contains the same active ingredient as the antidepressant medications WELLBUTRIN, WELLBUTRIN SR, and WELLBUTRIN XL."[14] And the FDA reiterates the fact that Zyban *is* an antidepressant when it further reports "Anyone considering the use of Zyban *or any other antidepressant…*" (italics mine)

The importance of having all the information about drugs hawked for alleged mental disorders cannot be understated when one considers the side effects associated with the antidepressant "treatment." The following are some of the known side effects of Wellbutrin/Zyban listed in the 2005 *Physicians Desk Reference (PDR)*: *agitation, abnormalities of mental status, neurological disturbances, mania/hypomania, hallucinations, depression, memory impairment, depersonalization, psychosis, mood instability, paranoia, formal thought disorder, suicidal ideation.* Sounds awful, and one might wonder how any one or number of these adverse effects is worse than smoking.

But what is interesting to note about the utilities of both Prozac/Sarafem and Wellbutrin/Zyban is that neither Eli Lilly nor GlaxoSmithKline conducted clinical trials comparing the effectiveness of the drugs for the alleged stated mental illness against the other. In other words, how would Prozac stack up against Sarafem in treating PMDD or Wellbutrin against Zyban in treating smoking cessation? One can only wonder about the outcomes of such trials. But given that there is no chemical difference between Prozac/Sarafem and Wellbutrin/Zyban one might expect similar if not identical clinical trial outcomes, further suggesting that the drugs do not target a specific alleged mental abnormality.

What is clear, though, despite the pharmaceutical sleight-of-hand, all of the above drugs, regardless of how they are marketed, are antidepressants and carry with them the FDA "black box" warning "Suicidal Thoughts or Actions in Children and Adults" (in part): "FDA is highlighting that adults being treated with antidepressant medication, particularly those being treated for depression, should be watched closely for worsening of depression and for increased suicidal thinking or behavior."[15]

The above warning is based on preliminary data and the FDA began a more comprehensive review in July 2005 to determine if the increased risk of suicidality is due to the antidepressant drugs. While it is anyone's guess when, or if, the FDA will complete its review of the adverse effects of antidepressants on adults, many within and outside of the medical community believe it is a forgone conclusion. There are abundant data available today and a great deal of information that has been around long before the approval of Prozac, that establishes a connection between psychiatric mind-altering antidepressants and suicide and other harmful, potentially deadly behaviors.

Regardless of what is thought or believed, the deep thinkers at the FDA went to medical school and, therefore, are fully aware that there is no psychiatric diagnosis that is a disease – an objective, confirmable abnormality of the brain— and also are fully aware that the above mentioned "treatments," Prozac/Sarafem, Wellbutrin/Zyban, regardless of how they are marketed, are identical chemical compounds. And they are aware that for more than two decades patients have been experiencing potentially life-threatening adverse reactions to antidepressant "treatments."

Given the above, it appears that Americans have not been given *all* the information they need and deserve in order to make informed decisions about either their alleged mental illness or their treatment options. This is no accident, and Dr. Breggin for decades, through his numerous books, has tried to make the facts available. In 1999 Breggin teamed with David Cohen, Ph.D., to write *Your Drug May be Your Problem; How and Why to Stop Taking Psychiatric*

Medications, which is a must-read for anyone interested in learning about psychiatric drugs. Breggin and Cohen provide good insight into how Americans became convinced of their mental illness and dependent on mind-altering drugs.

"It is all a matter of definition—of naming and labeling. When emotional discomfort or suffering is defined as a 'disorder,' it creates business for doctors and drug companies. The campaigns to promote 'mental illness' have been so successful that, within a matter of a few years, millions of Americans have come to believe that they have 'biochemical imbalances,' 'panic disorder,' or 'clinical depression,' and that their children have 'ADHD.'"

"As a result of successful marketing campaigns, consumers tend to identify trade names with generic products. We ask for Kleenex when we mean any brand of soft facial tissue. We ask for a Xeroxed copy when we mean a photocopy. And we speak of the "Prozac nation" when referring to antidepressants or even psychiatric drugs in general. There is hardly a person alive who doesn't experience moments or even hours and days of anxiety, depression, or other emotional "symptoms," making it easy for drug advocates to claim, for example, that half of all Americans will suffer a psychiatric disorder at some time in their lives. In actuality, however, these campaigns—including the ones directed to depression and anxiety— are stigmatizing and demoralizing people, who in turn, end up believing that they must have a mental illness."[16]

While Breggin and Cohen's characterization of psychiatric diagnosing being "stigmatizing" and "demoralizing" is accurate, given that the psychiatric community deceptively sells mental illness as disease and the pharmaceutical companies hawk virtually identical mind-altering drugs as "new" and targeting specific alleged mental abnormalities, the word "insulting" also comes to mind.

Preliminary FDA data suggest that American adults fair no better than America's children when it comes to experiencing adverse reactions to the psychiatric mind-altering drugs, and knowing which psychiatric patients may become victims of such events is anyone's guess. The fact remains that the drug companies and the FDA do not understand how the drugs work in the adult brain for a specific alleged mental illness anymore than they know how the drugs work on the adolescent brain. Neither does anyone in the psycho-pharmacological community know the cause(s) of any alleged psychiatric disorder. And, finally, the FDA has warned the adult population that these mind-altering drugs may cause suicidal ideation and other harmful behaviors.

Successful marketing and mental health information campaigns have convinced tens of millions of Americans that they suffer from diseases of the brain when there is no proof to substantiate these claims. In fact, quite the opposite is true and Breggin and Cohen in their book, *Your Drug May be Your Problem*, summed up the reality of psychiatric drugging this way: "In modern psychiatric treatment, we take the single most complicated known creation in the universe – the human brain – and pour drugs into it in the hope of "improving" its function when in reality we are disrupting its function."[17]

"Ironically," Breggin and Cohen conclude, "psychiatric drugs cause rather than cure biochemical imbalances in the brain. In fact, the only known biochemical imbalances in the brains of patients routinely seen by psychiatrists are brought about by the psychiatrists themselves through the prescription of mind-altering drugs. Psychiatric drugs "work" precisely by causing imbalances in the brain – by producing enough brain malfunction to dull the emotions and judgment or to produce an artificial high."[18]

This is information that the public will not find distributed by the pharmaceutical companies or the FDA, and because the public is mostly unaware of the other side of the psychiatric drug story, Americans have not been fully informed in order to make intelligent decisions about their mental health care.

Worse still, it appears that between the public's ignorance and the psycho-pharma industry's financial muscle, a sweeping Hitleresque initiative has begun nationwide that, when fully implemented, intends to subject every American to routine mental health exams, whether they want it or not.

[1] Food and Drug Administration Public Health Advisory, "Suicidality in Adults Being Treated with Antidepressant Medications," June, 30, 2005.

[2] Jeanne Lenzer., "FDA to Review "Missing" Drug Company Documents," *British Medical Journal* (BMJ) January 1, 2005.

[3] "U.K. Medical Journal Retracts Report on Missing Prozac Data," *Associated Press, Wall Street Journal, January 27, 2005.*

[4] Amanda Gardner, "Prozac Maker Knew of Problems in 1988," *HealthDayNews*, December 30, 2004.

[5] Kelly Patricia O'Meara, "Prettier In Pink: Eli Lilly Has Renamed Prozac And Is Selling It to Treat PMS/PMDD as 'Mental Illness,' *Insight* Magazine, April 30, 2001. pp-10-13.

[6] Peter R. Breggin, M.D., "An Examination of Eli Lilly Company's Contentions that the BMJ Prozac Documents were Never Missing and Have No Significance," January 12, 2005, pg-6.

[7] Ibid, Pg-5.

[8] Ibid, Pg-5.

[9] Eli Lilly and Company, "Conditions & Diseases" www.lilly.com/products/conditions/.

[10] Karl Loren, Prozac Petition "The Office of the Surgeon General of the United States; The Department of Health & Human Services; The Federal Bureau of Investigations and The Justice Department. Legal Law Help "Safety and Health," http://www.legallawhelp.com/safety_and_health/prozac/.

[11] United States Government Accountability Office, "Adverse Drug Events – The Magnitude of Health Risk is Uncertain Because of Limited Incidence Data," January 2000, pg-10.

[12] Thomas J. Moore, "Hard to Swallow," *Washingtonian Magazine*, December 1997.

[13] "Lilly Issues Response to British Medical Journal," Eli Lilly and Company, December 31, 2004.

[14] Food and Drug Administration, Prescribing Information, Zyban (Bupropion Hydrochloride), Pg-1.

[15] Food and Drug Administration, FDA Alert, "Suicidal Thoughts or Actions in Children and Adults," July 2005.

[16] Peter R. Breggin, M.D., David Cohen, Ph.D., "Your Drug May Be Your Problem: How and Why to Stop Taking Psychiatric Medications," Perseus Books, Reading Mass., Pg-90-91.

[17] Ibid., Pg-7.

[18] Ibid., Pg-41.

Chapter Seven

Something Wicked This Way Comes

The late president of the United States, Ronald Reagan, aptly explained government intervention this way: "The nine most terrifying words in the English language are, 'I'm from the government and I'm here to help.'" Nowhere is this quote more appropriate than when applied to George W. Bush's President's New Freedom Commission on Mental Health (NFC).

While the sweeping initiative has been sold as a benevolent effort to bring mental health care to all Americans, a cursory review reveals there is nothing "free" about the NFC's initiative, and upon closer examination it appears that the benevolence is directed at two groups that stand to profit from "a fundamental transformation of the nation's approach to mental health"—the psychiatric community and the pharmaceutical industry.

This is an especially important issue to follow when one recalls that in 2004 the FDA issued Public Health Warnings that SSRI/SNRI antidepressants may increase suicidal thoughts and other harmful behaviors in an unknown number of children and adults taking antidepressants—the mind-altering drugs of choice for "treating" alleged mental illnesses.

The NFC is part of Bush's support and commitment to screen all Americans for possible mental illnesses which, more likely than not, require treatment in the form of mind-altering drugs. Yes, that's right; apparently too many Americans are falling through the mental health cracks and not getting the help they need. By placing additional financial burdens on taxpayers—to the tune of hundreds of millions, if not billions, of dollars—to fund the programs, the president intends to *help* Americans by supporting newly created federal, state and local mental health programs, whether Americans want the help or not. The NFC's stated purpose is to ensure that mental illnesses are caught as early as possible in order that appropriate treatment—drugs—can be administered to allow long, happy and productive lives.

In light of the fact that psychiatric diagnoses are not based in science, and the mind-altering drugs used in treatment are potentially life-threatening to an unknown percentage of the population, saying that this kind of government help is Orwellian, extraordinarily intrusive and terrifying is putting it mildly.

The push to identify America's mentally ill began in April 2002 when Bush established the NFC, which was tasked with conducting a comprehensive study of the mental health service delivery system in the U.S. and, based on the findings, make recommendations how best to fix the system. Members of the NFC were to identify policies that could be implemented by federal, state and local governments to promote psychiatric screening, enhance utilization of treatment interventions and streamline delivery of medical services.

Minus all the we-want-to-help psycho-pharma language, what the initiative really is saying is through government financial support psychiatric diagnosing will be promoted, more children will be drugged and getting the drugs will be much easier. Bada-bing bada-boom!

The NFC Executive Summary delivered to Bush in July 2003 reads as if it were written by the psycho-wizards at the APA in conjunction with the pharmaceutical industry. For example, the NFC Executive Summary begins: "We envision a future when everyone with a mental illness will recover, a future when mental illnesses can be prevented or cured, a future when mental illnesses are detected early, and a future when everyone with a mental illness at any stage of life has access to effective treatment and supports—essentials for living, working, learning, and participating fully in the community."[1] Sounds patriotic, almost as if "God Bless America" is playing in the background, huh?

But what immediately comes to mind after reading the above NFC we're-looking-out-for-your-best-mental-health-interests opener is that it might be easier to swallow the benevolent grand plans for the nation's mental health if the commission first could cough up scientific and/or medical proof that any of the nearly 400 psychiatric diagnoses actually are objective, confirmable abnormalities of the brain. As has been demonstrated time and again throughout this book, having objective, confirmable science to support the mental "abnormality" is no impediment to planet psycho-pharma, as it has never depended on scientific discovery of diseases of the brain to make psychiatric diagnoses or to create mind-altering drugs to treat the alleged brain abnormalities.

But the NFC's chairman, Michael F. Hogan, director of the Ohio Department of Mental Health, further explains in the summary: "The Commission's findings confirm that there are unmet needs and that many barriers impede care for people with mental illnesses. Mental illnesses are shockingly common; they affect almost every American family."[2] "Shockingly common?" Is Hogan kidding?

Alleged mental illnesses are a dime a dozen and growing by leaps and bounds with every new printing of the APA's *Diagnostic and Statistical Manual* (*DSM*). In fact, based on the ever-increasing number of alleged mental disorders, the line between normal and abnormal behavior is becoming indistinguishable. If one is shy, sad, depressed, too happy, drinks or eats too much or too little, smokes, wiggles, doesn't pay attention, is forgetful or has any number of phobias, they can be diagnosed as suffering from a mental illness requiring psychiatric treatment in the form of drugs.

Given that there virtually is an alleged mental illness to fit every human emotion, the NFC's recommendations take on a whole new meaning in the organization's quest to help Americans. For example, the NFC recommends the following:

- Both children and adults **will be screened** for mental illnesses during their routine physical exams—across the lifespan. (Goal 4, page 11) (Emphasis added)

- Schools assist in screening: "All youngsters in a school to be screened for mental disorders… schools are in a key position to identify mental health problems early and to provide a link to appropriate services." (Goal 4, page 58)

- The early detection of mental health problems in children and adults—through routine and comprehensive testing and screening—will be an expected and typical occurrence. (Goal 4, page 11)

In order to carry out the grand nationwide psych plan for America's children, the NFC recommended to Bush that Columbia University's TeenScreen program be utilized for early intervention. The meat and potatoes of the TeenScreen program is to "ensure that all youth are offered a mental health check-up before graduating from high school." And, the further goal is to "identify and refer for treatment those who are at risk for suicide or suffer from an untreated mental illness."

The "features" that the TeenScreen program "offers" include:

- All youngsters in a school will be screened.
- Parental consent is required.
- Computer-based questionnaires will be used to screen for mental illness and suicide risk.
- Columbia University TeenScreen Program provides consultation, screening materials, software, training and technical assistance to qualifying schools and communities.
- In return, TeenScreen partners are expected to screen at least 200 youth per year and ensure that a licensed mental health professional is on site to give immediate counseling and referral services for youth at greatest risk.
- When the program identifies youth needing treatment, their care is paid for depending on the family's health coverage. (NFC Summary, page 63)

While the "features" of the plan sound good, a real desire to help America's suffering children, the devil most definitely is in the details. First, what is clear is that every American school-age child will be given a mental health exam, and this will be done, according to the plan, with parental consent. Well, that's not entirely true. The reality is much more devious.

The TeenScreen program uses two consent forms—active and passive. The active consent form requires that children have parents check "yes" or "no" if the child's participation in the mental health screening is approved or disapproved; then the form must be signed and returned to the school. The passive form (waiver of consent) requires that parents return the form only if they **do not want** their child to participate in the screening. In other words, if the parent fails to return the passive form their child will be screened—something along the lines of "Hey, you didn't return the form so we assume you want your kid's mental health tested."

This is an interesting concept when one considers the large number of children that may forget to return the signed "opt-out" form to the school. But the active/passive forms take on a whole new meaning when one further considers the caveat spelled out on the TeenScreen website:

"Protection of Pupil Rights Act (PPRA)"

PPRA is a federal law that protects the rights of parents by making instructional materials available for their inspection if the materials are to be used in connection with a survey, analysis or evaluation in which their child is participating and which is funded by the U.S. Department of Education. The law also requires written parental consent before minors are required to take part in such a survey, analysis, or evaluation.

*If your local mental health screening program is approved by the Board of Education as part of the educational program, **you are not required to get active parental consent** under PPRA. Passive consent is sufficient in this circumstance. It is best to recommend that, if passive consent is obtained from parents, then active consent **should be sought** from participants as a safeguard.*

Active parental consent must be obtained, however, if a child is going to be removed from an instructional activity for screening. However, if the screening will be given to all students, as opposed to some, it becomes part of the curriculum and no longer requires active parental consent (i.e., if all ninth-graders will be screened as a matter of policy, it is considered part of the curriculum).[3] (Emphasis added)

The gist of the above policy is that if the local board of education approves the program as part of the school curriculum, then parental consent is not required. And, although TeenScreen suggests obtaining active consent as a safeguard, the program only explains that it *"should"* be sought, not that it *"must"* be sought. Given the above, parents no longer have to be concerned only with the progress of their children's reading, writing and arithmetic abilities, they also have to be on a constant vigil, interrogating their child on a weekly basis about whether the school intends to test their child for alleged mental disorders.

This, of course, says nothing about the fear, confusion and anxiety elementary school children may experience waiting in line for tests which will determine whether they suffer from a mental illness—that's if the child even understands what it means to be labeled mentally ill, especially in later years like junior and senior high school.

More importantly, even though the initiative talks about ways to reduce the stigma associated with mental illness, one is compelled to consider how this is possible when being labeled with a mental illness—an alleged brain abnormality—is, in itself, stigmatizing. For instance, what happens when children become aware of a classmate's mental illness label, unless, of course, the plan is to slap a label on a majority of children, making the norm well…abnormal? Parents, though, are all too aware of how hurtful adolescents can be, and it seems fair to suggest that the future doesn't look emotionally promising for those children being labeled as mentally abnormal. Nevertheless, apparently ignoring these bothersome issues, the deep thinkers who concocted the grand mental health initiative decided it was in the best interest of America's children to move forward at all costs.

The first step in the grand mental health plan then is to obtain parental consent which, TeenScreen has made clear, is not mandatory in a number of scenarios. Step two is the first leg of the actual screening process. The TeenScreen program utilizes three "instruments" for determining the likelihood of a mental health "problem." The first "tool" that may be used in the screening process is the Columbia Health Screen (CHS), a 14-item self-completion questionnaire that takes about 10 minutes to complete.

The second "tool" that may be used for screening is the Columbia Depression Scale (CDS) consisting of 22 items that also is a self-completion, paper-and-pencil questionnaire. The CDS may not be quite as good as the CHS because the CDS can be completed in a record eight minutes. Both of the above self-completion screening tools are approved for 11- to 18-year-olds, and what will really impress and instill confidence in the screening process is that both the CDS and the CHS, which allegedly show the "likelihood" of a mental health problem with a child, can be scored by "trained non-professionals." That's right, if taken literally, the lunchroom personnel can be trained to score your child's mental health test!

The final "tool" available by TeenScreen to determine if a child is at risk of suffering from a mental illness is the Diagnostic Predictive Scales (DPS), which is a 52-item, computerized interview that also can be scored by "trained non-professionals." The DPS computer test is designed for 9- to 18-year-olds and also takes just 10 minutes, but this test produces a computer-generated report of the results.

Wow, that's impressive! Just answer a few questions and 10 minutes later a child may be a candidate for a psychiatric diagnosis. In fact, it appears that the TeenScreen process of determining which of America's children may be suffering from a mental illness is speedier than lunch-time ordering at most drive-thru fast-food restaurants!

Then again, speed is definitely something Americans crave, but is it such a good idea when it comes to deciding the mental health of the nation? There are clues provided by TeenScreen, though, that suggest that even the psycho-wizards who created the program know, no matter how speedy, the tests may not be appreciated by parents of America. This is evident by what is missing from the information provided at TeenScreen's website (http://www.teenscreen.org).

The entire program, of course, is about helping children who have fallen through the cracks, determining if they are suffering from some alleged mental illness but, oddly enough, TeenScreen does not post for informational review the specific questions from the tests that will be posed to the children. Why? Would not having all the information about the program help garner support and confidence from the masses? Although I have obtained copies of two of the tests, officials at TeenScreen did not respond to my request for reprint approval.

Given that all three tests involve questions, in part, that specifically deal with the child having thoughts about killing himself/herself; it is not difficult to understand why the questions have been withheld from public review. Really, one has to wonder how many parents would consider it a good idea for their 9-year-old elementary school child to be questioned about suicidal thoughts, how often they have the thoughts and if they've ever tried to kill themselves. It seems fair to say that there may not be a whole lot of parents pumped up about having their elementary school children even having to consider answers to such questions but, then again, given that many parents may not be aware that their child is taking the mental illness test, they'll only learn about the questions when the child is referred to Step Three.

The third step and, perhaps, the most liberal step in the screening process, consists of an interview with an on-site clinician, who will review the test score (which may have been scored by a trained non-professional) and then spend a "brief" amount of time talking with the child. In Step Three, the "on-site" clinician then will complete the "Screening Information Form," which consists of checking off in the positive or negative whether the child displays symptoms relating to alleged mental disorders such as social phobias, panic disorder, generalized anxiety, obsessive compulsive disorder, depression and suicide.

What extraneous questions may be posed to the child is anyone's guess. This particular point is of concern to many familiar with the grand mental health initiative, including Jane Orient, MD., executive director of the Association of American Physicians and Surgeons, who writes in part:

"Teams of experts are awaiting the infusion of cash. They'll be ensconced in your child's school before you even know it. A bonus is that your little darlings will probably give them quite a bit of information about you also, and then you, too, can receive therapy you didn't know you needed. Do you sometimes raise your voice? Ever spank them? Hug them inappropriately? Have politically incorrect attitudes? Use forbidden words? Own a gun? Smoke cigarettes, especially indoors? Read extremist literature? Refuse to recycle? Prepare for a knock on the door.

There are many tools at the disposal of the mental health squad. Counseling sessions; drugs (Ritalin, antidepressants, tranquilizers, maybe some new ones that need to be tested on some experimental subjects of your child's age); group therapy; removing the child from the home (this may be a "last resort," but often the mere threat can accomplish wonders.) Miraculously, throughout human history most of those crazy children have become stable, productive adults without federally mandated psychiatric treatment. Still more amazingly, their parents have managed also. Psychiatry in the hands of government, instead of independent physicians who are working for patients, reeks of Orwell's "1984" or the Soviet era." [4]

Beyond the vast number of unknowns associated with the sweeping mental health initiative, such as the issues raised by Dr. Orient and others, is the base-line problem. While the interview process sounds as if it is medically and scientifically based, the fact is all of the symptoms listed on the "Screen Information Form" are extracted from the symptoms listed in the *DSM-IV* published by the APA, and which are not based in science but rather are subjective criteria, essentially opinions, included in the *DSM* by a vote/ consensus by committees of psycho-wizards at the APA.

In other words, America's children will be diagnosed with mental disorders based on a subjective understanding of the answers provided to the clinician, and not based on any medical or scientific test such as an X-ray, CAT, MRI or PET scan, or blood test, and, as has been well-demonstrated throughout this book, there is no known objective, confirmable abnormality to prove a single psychiatric diagnosis.

Nevertheless, once the preliminary psychiatric diagnosis has been made by the on-site clinician (whoever that is and whatever extraneous information is pulled from the child about their home life) the parents then are contacted and "offered" assistance with obtaining services in the community. But what if the parents don't buy into the subjective diagnosis? What if parents of America tell the clinician to take the alleged mental illness and stick it in their ear?

It's as if a negative response from parents is not a consideration, and TeenScreen doesn't even address the issue of declining the "offered" help that wasn't initiated by the parents in the first place. But spending just a half an hour on the Internet reviewing gut-wrenching cases of families whose children have been removed or threatened with removal from the home by child welfare authorities because parents refused to drug their children may provide some indication of what lies ahead for parents who refuse the "offered" help.

Additionally, the November 2005 decision of the 9th U.S. Circuit Court of Appeals in California sheds further light on what parents may expect should they find the questions about sex and suicide posed to their young children offensive. In the Palmdale, Calif., school district, for purposes of research, children were surveyed about sex and suicidal thoughts. According to one boy, Jimmy Fields, who was 11 at the time of the survey, "They said well, they asked me how often I masturbate, how often do I think about killing myself, do I want to touch other people's private parts?..."[5] When parents got wind of the research, six of the families sued the Palmdale school district for robbing them of their constitutional right to control their children's upbringing, arguing that it is the parents decision to decide what is discussed with their children. The 9th Circuit Court of Appeals upheld a lower court decision and dismissed the families' lawsuit, finding that "parents do not have a fundamental right to be the exclusive providers of information of a sexual nature and that the survey was a reasonable state action."

Assuming that there may be many parents, like those above who are offended by the mental health questionnaires and decide to decline the "offered" help, what then happens to the information gathered during the screening and interview process? Who has access to the child's TeenScreen test results, other than the "trained non-professional" who scored the test and the "on-site" clinician? According to the TeenScreen website it really is anybody's guess:

"Screening personnel should determine with the school officials whether or not they are permitted access to student records without the formal consent of parents. Certain personnel may, however, be privy to the records under these exceptions: school officials with a legitimate education interest, organizations conducting certain studies for or on behalf of the school and appropriate officials in the case of health and safety emergencies." [6]

What is a "legitimate education interest," which organizations conducting what studies and what health and safety emergencies? TeenScreen does not offer specifics to the above, and the criteria are so broad that one seriously has to wonder who won't be privy to the child's personal mental health information. This is an interesting concept when one recalls that information about what psychiatric drugs school shooters may have been prescribed is handled as if it were a state secret.

Okay, time for a recap. According to the TeenScreen website, parents do not have to provide consent for their child to be screened for a mental illness, a "trained non-professional" can score the tests and it is anyone's guess just who will have access to the child's mental illness diagnosis. And, the crescendo, of course, is that all of this psychiatric diagnosing is based on subjective non-scientific criteria, which was voted into existence by a consensus of the deep thinkers at the APA. What, the help doesn't sound too good? It gets worse.

Once the child has completed the screening process, parents then are notified and "offered" assistance with getting help for their suffering child in the mental health community—in other words, a psychiatric referral. What is interesting to note on the TeenScreen website is the attention given to the importance of diagnosing children who may be suicidal. All kinds of facts and figures are provided by the program to support the need for early diagnosis of mental illnesses that may lead to suicide, and TeenScreen reports: "Research has shown that a significant association exists between these disorders and suicide risk."[7]

While TeenScreen would have America believe that screening a school-age child will somehow deter the child from future suicidal thoughts and actions, this is at odds with other expert opinions. For instance, the U.S. Preventive Services Task Force (USPSTF) an independent panel of experts in primary care and prevention that systematically reviews the evidence of effectiveness and develops recommendations for clinical preventive services, gives suicide screening its lowest recommendation: (in part)

"The USPSFT found no evidence that screening for suicide risk reduces suicide attempts or mortality. There is limited evidence on the accuracy of screening tools to identify suicide risk in the primary care setting, including tools to identify those at high risk. The USPSTF found insufficient evidence that treatment of those at high risk reduces suicide attempts or mortality. The USPSTF found no studies that directly address the harms of screening and treatment of suicide risk. As a result, the USPSFT could not determine the balance of benefits and harms of screening for suicide risk in the primary care setting."[8]

So, according to the USPSFT, there is insufficient evidence to support the claim that screening reduces the risk of suicide attempts, and it further states that there is insufficient evidence that "treatment" reduces suicide attempts. This is important information when one considers the other goal associated with the nationwide mental health plan. Although the TeenScreen program is about screening the children of America for mental illness and getting those at risk the help they need, TeenScreen claims that the "program does not involve treatment and does **not** recommend or endorse any particular kind of treatment for the youth who are identified by the screening."

It is true that TeenScreen does not recommend the specific treatment the children may be prescribed, but TeenScreen clearly is an advocate of increased drugging, and the point is well made by the director of TeenScreen, Laurie Flynn, whose cozy relationship with the psychiatric community and pharmaceutical industry will be explored later in this chapter, when she wrote "the long-term goal of TeenScreen is not just identification, but treatment for those in need."[9]

So, according to the director of TeenScreen, getting America's children treatment is the "long-term goal." But what are the treatments for the alleged mental illnesses for which children will be screened, such as depression, social phobias, panic disorders, anxiety and obsessive compulsive disorders? That's right, psychiatric mind-altering drugs, the very drugs that effectively have been banned for adolescent use in the United Kingdom and more than two-dozen other nations in the European Union. Closer to home the FDA, so concerned about the adverse effects associated with antidepressants, requested that the pharmaceutical companies place "black box" warnings on the drugs.

The goal of TeenScreen is to treat America's children for mental illnesses that are not based in science with mind-altering drugs that even the pharmaceutical companies openly admit they do not know how the drugs work in the brain for the alleged mental illness and, worse still, may cause the very behaviors they allege to treat and, in fact, are potentially deadly. And, the kicker to the above is that the prescribing of mind-altering drugs will be done by primary care physicians, most of which are not trained, nor possess any expertise, in psychiatric diagnosing. But the NFC apparently took this into consideration and recommended an all-encompassing treatment plan that first was put into practice in Texas, under then-Governor George W. Bush's leadership.

The NFC recommended the Texas Medication Algorithm Project (TMAP) because "it illustrates an evidence-based practice that results in better consumer outcomes, including reduced symptoms, fewer and less severe side effects, and improved functioning."[10] But what exactly is a medication algorithm? Well, in a nutshell, it's a no-hassle, step-by-step flowchart used by physicians to decide what treatment (read: drugs) to prescribe to Americans allegedly suffering from mental illnesses. The medication algorithm requires that doctors follow specified treatment patterns.

One example of the medication algorithm is found in the treatment procedure for depression. According to TMAP, "Strategies for the Treatment of Major Depression" (Non-psychotic), includes seven stages containing what appear to be magic formulas to psychiatric wellness. The stages are as follows:

STAGE 1: Monotherapy (single drug): the physician may choose one mind-altering drug from the approved SSRIs (Prozac, Paxil, Zoloft or Celexa), or prescribe another antidepressant not specifically a SSRI, such as Wellbutrin, Serzone, Effexor or Remeron.

STAGE 2: Monotherapy (single drug): the physician may choose any one of the mind-altering drugs listed in Stage 1 or may choose a tricyclic antidepressant (TCA) such as Tofranil, Anafranil, Norpramin, Pamelor or Elavil (all of which are also sedatives).

STAGE 3: <u>Monotherapy</u> (single drug): the physician may choose one mind-altering drug listed in Stages 1 and 2, a tricyclic antidepressant or an MAOI (Monoamine Oxidase Inhibitor) including Nardil, Parnate and Marplan.

STAGE 4: <u>Augmentation</u>: The physician may prescribe any untried mind-altering antidepressant not listed in Stages 1,2 & 3 plus lithium, thyroid medication (Cytomel), or buspirone (BuSpar) simultaneously.

STAGE 5: <u>Combination Therapy</u>: The physician may prescribe a tricyclic antidepressant with an SSRI or choose the following combinations that must be taken simultaneously including, Wellbutrin plus an SSRI, or Serzone with a SSRI, or Wellbutrin with Serzone.

STAGE 6: <u>ECT: (Electroconvulsive Therapy "Electric Shock")</u>: If patient refuses ECT or does not respond, go to next stage or repeat an earlier stage with a different agent (drug).

STAGE 7: <u>Other</u>: Any antidepressant or combination not previously tried.

It is difficult to know where to begin when addressing the TMAP and how the NFC possibly could conclude the algorithm is the best course of action when it comes to treatment for the alleged psychiatric mental illnesses from which the nation's adult population is suffering, let alone its children. A good place to start may be in first acknowledging that there is no scientific method in which physicians can determine the level of any person's depression because there is no objective, confirmable abnormality found in the human brain that is depression.

Do children get depressed? Yes, of course. But can the level of depression be objectively measured? No. The level of depression is based on a subjective understanding of answers provided in response to questions posed by the physician and, worse still, there is no way for the physician to know what the patient's brain chemical levels are—and whether they are in or out of balance. This is a key point given that the algorithm "treatment" involves mind-altering drugs that increase the levels of naturally occurring chemicals in the brain.

But, even more odd, there is absolutely no discussion by the psycho-wizards at the APA or the pharmaceutical companies about the possibility that the "chemical imbalance," which supposedly would work both ways, may involve a person having too much of the naturally occurring chemical. And, if this is so, then increasing the levels of chemicals in a person who has too much of a specific brain chemical could produce some devastating effects. In other words, are people suffering because they have too little or too much of a brain chemical? Today, the pharmaceutical companies earn billions of dollars in revenues by suggesting people suffer from a deficit of a particular brain chemical and the "treatment" will increase the chemical levels. But what if the opposite is true? What if people actually suffer from having too much of a brain chemical? But, again, this is where science – objective, confirmable proof of a chemical imbalance – would come in handy.

But what should really twist some parental pantyhose is the algorithm itself. It is one thing for adults to make informed decisions and submit themselves to such chemical experiments but quite another when it comes to kids. It seems fair to say that when fully implemented, versions of the TMAP algorithm will become a national drug experiment; a nationwide pharmacological clinical trial, and America's children will become the unsuspecting participants/victims.

Based on the adult version of the TMAP, let's review a scenario that may be representative of what America's children will have to endure if subjected to a similar algorithm. A child is diagnosed with an alleged psychiatric mental illness and the physician is instructed to follow the algorithm chart of treatments. So, in the first stage, a mind-altering antidepressant is prescribed and, in some arbitrary amount of time, if there is no improvement of the alleged psychiatric mental illness, the child is moved to Stage 2.

In Stage 2, the child is taken off the first mind-altering antidepressant and prescribed a different mind-altering antidepressant or some other mind-altering drug that is non-SSRI/SNRI. Okay, darn, neither stage 1 or 2 helped the kid, back to the drawing board. The physician moves on to Stage 3 of the algorithm, which consists of changing the mind-altering antidepressant again or moving to some other mind-altering drug. Assuming that after receiving the mind-altering drugs offered in the first three stages there is some semblance of the child who first walked into the doctor's office; the physician now is really cooking and decides to move to Stage 4.

In this stage the physician is allowed to shake up things a bit and use a number of mind-altering drugs simultaneously, including prescribing any of the antidepressants listed for use in Stages 1, 2 or 3 that haven't already been tried and then throwing in some other mind-altering drugs outside the antidepressant class.

Still not working? No problem. Stage 5 offers the physician the opportunity to really experiment. That's right, in this stage, combinations or drug "cocktails" are utilized. The physician may prescribe any combination of the SSRIs and SNRIs with non-SSRIs/SNRIs. If the child survives what can only be described as a chemical lobotomy between Stages 1 through 5 and still isn't "better," the physician may move to the creepiest of the algorithm stages.

In Stage 6 a physician may offer the crème de la crème of psychiatric experimentation: electroshock therapy (ECT). Given that an extraordinarily large amount of electricity is passed through the brain—leaving many patients with little mental ability, intelligence or memory—one has to question what exactly is therapeutic about this monstrous procedure. And, of course, this procedure is conducted after the patient has experienced the equivalent of a chemical lobotomy.

Finally, though, if the ECT is declined, Stage 7 leaves the physician the last resort, returning to Stage 1 and again prescribing more antidepressants or combinations of mind-altering drugs that have yet to be tried. As there are more than 30 antidepressants on the market, it appears that the physician could be busy for months or years experimenting with various drug cocktail combinations, certain to increase pharmaceutical company coffers but leaving America's children mentally bankrupt, which the psychiatric community will blame on the "underlying" mental illness.

Recall that the mind-altering drugs that will be prescribed in the algorithm as "treatment" effectively are banned for use in children by most of the nations that make up the European Union, and here in the U.S. the FDA has warned the public—children and adults—that antidepressants "may increase suicidal thoughts and actions." The pharmaceutical companies acknowledge that adverse reactions to the antidepressant drugs include mania, suicidal thoughts, hyperactivity, psychosis, hallucinations, confusion, anxiety and depression. Considering the above, it's as if the benevolent ones sitting on the NFC had lost all sense of logic and reason and still recommended the TMAP as the standard, despite the fact that many of the mind-altering drugs intended for use in the algorithm have *not* been approved for adolescent use. Still hearing "God Bless America" in the background?

Clearly, early intervention of America's children is a road paved in mind-altering drugs and yet, Laurie Flynn, director of Columbia University's TeenScreen, testified before Congress in March 2004 proudly describing the progress being made in saving America's suffering children. "In 2003, we were able to screen approximately 14,200 teens at these sites; among those students, we were able to identify approximately 3,500 youth with mental health problems and link them with treatment." And, apparently beaming with pride over the numbers of children they have been able to identify and "treat," Flynn further laid out for Congress the program's future dreams: "This year, we believe we will be able to identify close to 10,000 teens in need, a 300 percent increase over last year."[11]

But it got worse when Flynn further testified that "the need for increased screening is evidenced by the fact that close to 750,000 teens are depressed at any one time, and an estimated 7 million to 12 million youth suffer from mental illness. While treatments are available for these severely disabling disorders, sadly, most children do not receive the treatment they need. Among teens that are depressed, 60-80 percent go untreated."[12]

Is it really a "fact" that 750,000 teens are depressed? How long are they depressed and why. And, who makes the subjective diagnosis?

Flynn did not provide Congress with any objective, confirmable proof that depression is an abnormality of the brain, nor did she provide objective, confirmable proof that the "treatments"—mind-altering drugs—target a specific depression center in the brain. Yet, the TeenScreen advocate says it's a "fact" that so many hundreds-of-thousands of children are depressed. Ugh!

Beyond these very obvious and terribly important points, anyone who covers this issue regularly might be interested in knowing what number of the 3,500 youth the TeenScreen program identified as having mental illnesses previously had been diagnosed with another alleged mental disorder and had been prescribed mind-altering drugs. In other words, how many of the 3,500 had earlier been diagnosed with an alleged mental illness like ADHD and had been prescribed Ritalin, Adderall or Strattera, or any number of mind-altering drugs?

Flynn, like so many of the deep thinkers involved in the national initiative to mass identify and treat Americans for mental illness, has an impressive history with the pharmaceutical industry, having spent nearly two decades as the executive director of the National Alliance for the Mentally Ill (NAMI), the lobbying organization that boasts it is "The Nation's Voice on Mental Illness." During Flynn's 16-year tenure as NAMI's director, the lobbying organization received tens of millions of dollars from the pharmaceutical industry, many of which produce the very same mind-altering drugs that have been recommended for utilization in the flowchart algorithms, including the makers of the antidepressant Prozac (Eli Lilly and Co.) and the cocaine-like treatment for ADHD, Ritalin (Novartis Pharmaceuticals).

Many may accurately conclude that it was Flynn's exemplary work at NAMI that helped her land the top spot at TeenScreen, and even Flynn admits that NAMI long has been an integral part of the mass mental health initiative, acknowledging: "The TeenScreen Program developed 10 years ago by Columbia University and *offered in partnership with the National Alliance for the Mentally Ill* helps communities across the nation identify teens with mental illness who might be at risk for suicide."[13] (italics mine)

What is of additional interest is the extraordinary pharmaceutical support provided during the process of formulating the TMAP, which will be utilized once the mental illness diagnosis has been made. Allen Jones, an investigator in the Commonwealth of Pennsylvania Office of the Inspector General, Bureau of Special Investigations, is intimately familiar with the pharmaceutical power behind TMAP, and alleges in a whistleblower lawsuit that he was wrongfully removed from his investigation for his attempts to expose evidence of major pharmaceutical wrongdoing during his investigation of the Model Program being implemented in Pennsylvania. During his investigation, Jones uncovered the following:

1. This consortium sought to "legitimize" the medications recommended in the model program's "drug menus." The group elected to utilize "Expert Consensus Guidelines," rather than clinical studies or drug trials to form these recommendations.

2. Essentially, TMAP opted to "establish" new drugs as the best drugs for various illnesses by surveying the opinions of doctors and psychiatrists of TMAP's own choosing. **No hard science, no patients, no study review, and no clinical trials**—just the "Expert Opinions" of persons TMAP elected to survey.

3. TMAP formulated the questions to be posed to these physicians and formulated the structure of the responses permitted. No input aside from the survey questions was solicited. A total of only **fifty-seven** doctors and psychiatrists responded to the medication survey.

4. TMAP independently analyzed the resultant responses.

5. The drug companies involved in financing and/or directly creating and marketing TMAP include: Janssen Pharmaceutica, Johnson & Johnson, Eli Lilly, AstraZeneca, Pfizer, Novartis, Janssen-Ortho-McNeil, GlaxoSmithKline,

Abbott, Bristol Myers Squibb, Wyeth-Ayerst, Forest Laboratories and U.S. Pharmacopeia.

6. Janssen was the most aggressive of the companies in developing this model and in directly compromising and influencing public officials. All of the other companies mentioned contributed funding to the effort.

7. The patented mental health drugs embedded within this model program include: Risperdal, Zyprexa, Seroquel, Geodone, Depakote, Paxil, Zoloft, Celexa, Wellbutrin, Zyban, Remeron, Serzone, Effexor, BuSpar, Adderall and Prozac, all manufactured by the above companies.

8. TMAP concluded that the atypical antipsychotic medications Risperdal, produced by Janssen Pharmaceutica, Zyprexa produced by Eli Lilly, and Seroquel, produced by AstraZeneca, are the drugs of choice for all first, second and third-line treatments for Schizophrenia.

9. TMAP concluded that all newer, patented antidepressants were superior to generics.

10. TMAP concluded that the patented bi-polar drugs were superior to generic drugs.[14]

Jones concludes his nearly 70-page report with a damning assessment of the unholy alliance between the pharmaceutical industry and political entities, saying: *"The pharmaceutical industry has methodically compromised our political system at all levels and has systematically infiltrated the mental health service delivery system of this nation. They are poised to consolidate their grip via the New Freedom Commission and the Texas Medication Algorithm Project. The pervasive manipulation of clinical trials, the non-reporting of negative trials and the cover-up of debilitating and deadly side effects render meaningful informed consent impossible by persons being treated with these drugs. Doctors and patients alike have been betrayed by the governmental entities and officials who are supposed to protect them.* "[15]

Jones is another in a long line who have come to the same conclusions about the psycho-pharma alliance, and even the most hardened advocates of the mass psycho-pharma screening initiative must acknowledge that the pharmaceutical companies have played a substantial role in the structuring of the TMAP and will reap an extraordinary financial windfall from the mass identification and treatment of America's alleged mentally ill.

Given that there is no science behind the identification madness, it's a simple equation: get diagnosed, get drugged. It is no secret that the psychiatric mind-altering drugs are becoming the bread-and-butter of pharmaceutical revenues. For instance, in 2003, Medco Health Solutions reported that the use of behavioral (psychiatric) drugs for children topped all other types of drugs at 17 percent of total spending, and in the same years, IMS Health (a market research firm) reported sales of antidepressants just under $20 billion, up 10 percent from 2002.

More importantly, though, unless they have been living in a tuna can, these same advocates must also consider the harmful and potentially deadly effects associated with such an experimental drugging initiative. Virtually all of the psychiatric "antidepressant" drugs recommended by the TMAP algorithm (the standard for all algorithms), according to the FDA, "may increase the risk of suicidal thinking and behavior."

Worse than that, the FDA's own review of the antidepressant drugs found that the placebo (sugar pill) was as effective as the mind-altering drugs in a majority of drugs under review. And psychiatric drugging of children has become so profitable that drug companies have stepped up marketing strategies for this age group and it now is the fastest-growing form of intervention for children. According to one research report, in 1996 600,000 prescriptions for Prozac alone were written for kids under the age of 18 and 203,000 for children between the ages of 6 and 12. But the height of insanity is the following figure: **Three thousand scripts were written for infants under the age of one!**[16] And, these numbers reflect prescriptions for mind-altering antidepressants that the FDA has ***not*** approved for adolescent use.

Sound crazy? Yes, but this is reality on planet psycho-pharma when the drug companies, in conjunction with the wizards of psychiatry, have tens of billions of dollars in drug sales on the line. Yes, apparently, the not walking or talking infants, whose brains quite literally still are developing, allegedly can be diagnosed with some mental illness requiring a psychiatric mind-altering drug as "treatment." Wouldn't one love to be a fly on the wall during that diagnosing session!

But like the people who want to believe that the "chemical imbalance" is a proven cause for psychiatric diagnoses, there are skeptics that still believe the grand plans for mass diagnosing of America is a good idea. Naturally, anything is possible, but what do the deep thinkers in mental health think of the plans that have been implemented so far? Michael Hogan, the NFC chairman and director of the Ohio Department of Mental Health (which utilized a TMAP-based medication algorithm) and recipient of the Eli Lilly Lifetime Achievement Award, provides interesting insight.

According to a *Columbus Dispatch* series titled "Drugged into Submission" that reported on the increased use of psychiatric drugs on babies; "Nearly 40,000 Ohio children on Medicaid were taking drugs for anxiety, depression, delusions, hyperactivity and violent behavior as of July (2004)." The article further reported that 696 Ohio children, ranging in age from newborns to 3 years old, received sedatives and powerful, mood-altering, mental health drugs…"[17] The *Dispatch* reports Hogan's view: "The biggest public-health crisis facing the state and nation is the number of children with mental illness who fail to receive any care of treatment. It's true children are more likely to get medication than counseling or other behavioral therapy if they go to their pediatrician or family doctor. But at the end of the day, meds are quite safe and effective."

The word "clueless" comes to mind when considering Hogan's "meds are quite safe and effective" response. Given that the FDA and health organizations around the world have either effectively banned the use of mind-altering psychiatric drugs for children or, at a minimum, posted public warnings about their potential for suicide and other harmful behaviors for those taking the drugs, Hogan's response that "meds are quite safe and effective" seems ignorant.

But Hogan's support of the drug flowchart algorithm appears to waiver when it becomes apparent that the mass-drugging plan sharply increased the state's Medicaid budget. During an interview on a local Ohio radio station, WIMA-AM, Hogan had this to say about Ohio's version of TMAP (OMAP): "Frankly it didn't work very well for us and we've discontinued it...increasingly it's clear that the scientists don't have pretty good information to give the doctors about which works best...so we thought, and frankly I thought at one point in time that this kind of algorithm where you'd give the docs, 'Try this first, try this second,' would be a good idea but it just hasn't worked that well."[18]

While many may see this reversal as a grand victory that the drugging program failed in Ohio, one cannot help but wonder how many children had participated in the "try this first, try this second" algorithm, and just how many mind-altering drugs Ohio adolescents were subjected to before it was decided that the step-by-step drugging plan wasn't working. But Hogan isn't the only one involved in the grand psycho-pharma plan who has interesting things to say about important elements of the national psych plan and, in fact, the creator of TeenScreen, psychiatrist David Shaffer, professor of child psychiatry at Columbia University and director, Division of Child Psychiatry, New York State Psychiatric Institute, admits mistakes can be made.

During an interview for *Trends in Evidence Based Neuropsychiatry (TEN)*, Shaffer had this to say about the accuracy of screening children for mental illnesses: "We did studies to look at the accuracy of the TeenScreen. What we found was that the TeenScreen approach misses hardly anybody, but it does identify a whole bunch of kids who aren't really suicidal, so you get a lot of false positives. And that means if you're running a large program at a school, you're going to cripple the program because you're going to have too many kids you have to do something about."[19]

Okay, let's recap. TeenScreen is so comprehensive that "it misses hardly anybody," but it also identifies "a whole bunch of kids who aren't suicidal?" What Shaffer is saying is that the psych tests do not provide accurate diagnoses'. If this doesn't have parents of America banging their heads on the kitchen table, what will? And the absurdity of the mental health screening initiative is made even more clear by TeenScreen guru Shaffer when he reports in his own 2004 study: "The CSS' positive predictive value of 16 percent (determined by a weighted prevalence of DISC positive in the sample) would result in 84 non-suicidal teens being referred for further evaluation for every 16 youths correctly identified." [20]

Since when does an 84 percent failure rate equate to a reliable scientific test? In other words, based on Shaffer's study of his own test, 84 students out of 100 will be incorrectly identified as suffering from a specific mental illness. One has to wonder if parents of America are informed of this astonishing statistic as part of the information to consider when having to decide whether or not to allow the mental health screening test. The TeenScreen program has been implemented in specific locations in nearly all 50 states and, yet, a review of five TeenScreen participation parent consent forms for the mental health screening in various towns in Florida, Indiana, New Jersey, Ohio and Missouri make no mention of the psych-screen failure rate. Oh, yeah, that sounds like informed consent!

In the end, though, Americans should be asking one question: What part of the mass nationwide mental health initiative has shown real success rates? One only need consider the increased psychiatric drug use to answer that question. The entire national psych-scheme is built on a scientifically unproven theory that the alleged psychiatric mental disorders are actual abnormalities of the brain and that chemical intervention (mind-altering drugs) targets the abnormalities. So, with help from the psychiatric community in screening Americans for mental illness, the use of psychiatric mind-altering drugs most assuredly will increase. Enter the pharmaceutical companies.

According to a report from Business Communications Co. Inc., specialists in technical-market research and industry analysis, in 2002 the global market value for prescription central nervous system (CNS) psychotherapeutic drugs was $32 billion, and pharmaceutical revenues for the CNS class is expected to increase to $45 billion by 2007, with the U.S. comprising nearly 65 percent of the global market.[21]

The above projections for pharmaceutical revenues leaves little doubt about America's insatiable appetite for mind-altering drugs and, if the adolescent screening initiative is as successful as TeenScreen director Flynn, believes, America's children will be responsible for much of the anticipated growth in pharmaceutical revenues. Data in the trends of psychotropic drug users provided by Express Scripts Inc., a leading pharmacy benefit provider (not including Medicaid data), paints a clear picture of where the drugging is headed. Express Scripts reported in 2003 that in a five-year period (1998-2002) the use of antidepressants in children increased from 1.6 per 100 to 2.4 per 100—an adjusted annual increase of 9.2 percent, with the fastest-growing segment of users being preschoolers (newborns to 5 years old)..[22]

As a follow up to the FDA's revelations about the adverse effects associated with antidepressants, Express Scripts updated its study, reporting "the prevalence of antidepressant use in children continued to rise through the first half of 2004. The overall rate of antidepressant use in children grew from 1.47 percent in the first quarter of 2003 to 1.61 percent in first quarter 2004, a 9.4 percent increase in the prevalence of use. The growth in the rate of use was primarily driven by teenagers age 10–14 and 15–19."[23]

While there was a 20 percent drop in the use of mind-altering drugs immediately following the FDA's warnings about suicide associated with antidepressant use, it is doubtful that the drop will continue, especially in light of the efforts of TeenScreen. For example, out of 350 high school students screened by TeenScreen in Colorado, 87 percent of those tested were found to be either at risk of suicide or had a history of suicidal ideation. And, at Colorado youth homeless shelters, 71 percent screened positive for a psychiatric disorder.[24]

Does the word "absurd" come to mind? What TeenScreen would have us believe is that out of 350 high school students tested in Colorado, there were only 40 or so students who *weren't* thinking about suicide and, in homeless shelters, there only were 29 children out of a hundred not suffering from a mental disorder? And, recall, all of these impressive screening numbers are regurgitated as success stories in spite of TeenScreen's creator, Shaffer, admitting in his own study that there was an 84 percent failure rate—that only 16 children out of 100 were correctly identified.

But the implications of the above "success" rate in Colorado are truly Orwellian when one considers that there are 19.8 million 14- to 19-year-old children in the U.S. The grand psych plan is to screen each one for mental illnesses. If the same Colorado "success" rate (87 percent) is attained, the nation could have more than 17 million mentally ill teenagers being treated with potentially life-threatening mind-altering drugs.

Something wicked this way comes.

[1] Michael F. Hogan, Ph.D., Chairman, President's New Freedom Commission on Mental Health, Summary Cover Letter, July 22, 2003.

[2] Ibid. Pg-1.

[3] The TeenScreen News, Mental Health Check-ups For Youth, "Protection of Pupil Rights Act (PPRA), Fall 2003.

[4] Jane Orient, M.D., Outside View: Are your children crazy? *United Press International,* December 15, 2004.

[5] John Hattori, NBC News San Francisco, MSNBC Transcript, November 4, 2005

[6] The TeenScreen News, Mental Heatlh Check-ups For Youth, Volume 2, Issue 2, Fall 2003.

[7] TeenScreen, Columbia University, "Setting the Record Straight About TeenScreen," October 17, 2005.

[8] "Screening for Suicide Risk: Recommendation Statement; U.S. Preventive Services Task Force, May 2004.

[9] Laurie Flynn, *Community Voices* "Before Their Time: Preventing Teen Suicide," September 2005.

[10] Michael F. Hogan, Ph.D., Chairman, President's New Freedom Commission on Mental Health, Summary July 22, 2003, Pg-68.

[11] Laurie Flynn, Director, TeenScreen, Columbia University, U.S. Senate Committee on Health, Education, Labor, & Pensions, Congressional Testimony, "Suicide Prevention and Youth: Saving Lives," March 2, 2004

[12] Ibid.

[13] Laurie Flynn, *Community Voices* "Before Their Time: Preventing Teen Suicide," September 2005.

[14] Allen Jones, "Introduction" Law Project for Psychiatric Rights, January 20, 2004

[15] Allen Jones, "Rx:Smoke and Mirrors – The Texas Medication Algorithm Project," Law Project for Psychiatric Rights, January 20, 2004, pg 6-8.

[16] Barry Duncan, PSY.D., Scott Miller, PhD., and Jacqueline Sparks, MS, "The Myth of the Magic Pill," undated.

[17] Encarnacion Pyle, "Even Babies Getting Treated as Mentally Ill: Prescriptions on the rise even though they haven't been tested on children," *The Columbus Dispatch*, April 25, 2005.

[18] Michael Hogan, on-air Interview WIMA-AM Radio, Lima, Ohio, November 16, 2005.

[19] David Shaffer, F.R.C. Psych.., The Ten Interview, *Trends in Evidence-Based Neuropsychiatry*, March 2003.

Kelly Patricia O'Meara

David Shaffer, F.R.C. Psych. (Lond), Michelle Scott, Ph.D., Holly Wilcox, M.S., Carey Maslow, Ph.D., Roger Hicks, B.A., Christopher P.Lucas, M.D., Robin Garfinkel, Ph.D., and Steven Greenwald, M.A., "The Columbia SuicideScreen: Validity and Reliability of a Screen for Youth Suicide and Depression*," Journal of the American Academy of Child and Adolescent Psychiatry*, January 2004.

[21] Malika Rajan, "Global Market Value for Prescription Central Nervous System Psychotherapeutic Drugs to Reach Nearly $45 Billion by 2007," Business Communications Company, Inc., June 4, 2003.

[22] Express Scripts Inc., Research Study Findings, "Prevalence of Antidepressant Use in Children: 2003-2004."

[23] Ibid.

[24] Mental Health Association of Colorado, "Colorado Link Teen Violence & Suicide Prevention Project, 2003 www.mhacolorado.org/

Chapter Eight

The Fourth Estate:
The Blind Leading the Blind

Alert the media! Get Mike Wallace on the phone! Tom Cruise was right! Yes, it's a tough pill to swallow having a Hollywood superstar set the psychiatric record straight, but the fact is regardless of whether or not America appreciated the actor's passionate delivery during the June 2005 tit-for-tat between *Today Show* host Matt Lauer and Cruise, the actor's message was right on the money.

The Cruise-Lauer interview is a good example of why the public largely remains uninformed and misinformed about the fraud of psychiatric diagnosing and the dangers associated with mind-altering psychiatric drugs. More often than not, the nation's press corps provides an inaccurate, one-sided view of the psycho-pharma debate and, to the detriment of the public, regurgitates information provided by the psychiatric community as fact that, in reality, cannot be substantiated by science.

Rather than take advantage of the very public entrée to dig into the issue and provide an accurate, investigative, review of Cruise's comments about psychiatric diagnosing, with few exceptions the main stream media inexplicably took it as a green light to ridicule the actor about his spirituality, his delivery and the alleged inaccuracy of his comments.

The confrontational *Today* interview, for example, was covered by *New York Daily News* reporter Tracy Connor who wrote Cruise was "...pompously lecturing Matt Lauer about the evils of psychiatry— and scolding actress Brooke Shields for taking anti-depressants."[1]

If Connor had conducted even a cursory review of just one of Cruise's comments during the interview, such as "There is no such thing as a chemical imbalance" [in the brain], it seems fair to say that the derogatory spin might have been left out of the news piece and the

163

public might have gained insight into a potentially life-threatening issue. After all, the facts are not a state secret and as it has been well-established throughout this book by numerous respected doctors and researchers, there *is* no such thing as a "chemical imbalance" being the cause of any psychiatric disorder because there is no method to measure the chemical levels in the living human brain.

In other words, since there is no known method to measure the chemical levels in a living brain it is impossible to know whether an individual's brain chemistry is out of balance, or even what are the correct chemical levels. Whether the APA, the NIMH or the pharmaceutical companies *believe* alleged mental illnesses are caused by a chemical imbalance in the brain, believing, hoping and wishing, by any stretch of the imagination, are not scientific standards and do not equate objective, confirmable abnormality.

In the same article, Connor further pushes to discredit Cruise's remarks by bringing in the planet psycho-pharma power hitters to comment: "His proselytizing is also angering psychiatrists, who fear the Hollywood top gun could undo decades of work to remove the stigma from mental illness and psychiatric treatment." Dr. John Scully, medical director of the APA, is quoted in Connor's article saying: "The illnesses we treat—anxiety, depression—are very real illnesses.... The treatments work. We have demonstrated that through robust scientific study."

Nothing like stating the obvious. Who doesn't believe that anxiety and depression are "real" and also would not acknowledge that these emotional states have been around since the time of Adam and Eve. But that wasn't what was being debated. The debate was about the pseudoscience (subjectivity) that is psychiatric diagnosing and whether the alleged mental illnesses are due to objective, confirmable abnormalities ("chemical imbalances") of the brain.

The crescendo, though, is Connor's opinion of Cruise's remarks. She wrote that they are "void of scientific proof," following up her opinion with Scully's nonsensical summation: "It's a little like talking to somebody who claims the world is flat."

The response provided by the APA's mouthpiece does not contradict what the actor said but, rather, is further proof that the psychiatric organization so completely believes it has hoodwinked the American public that if anyone, especially one of those Hollywood star types, challenges the organization's unscientific claims they must be suffering from some kind of mental deficit, something along the lines of the alleged mental disorder oppositional defiant disorder (ODD).

The fact is Connor may believe that Cruise's comments are "devoid of scientific proof," which would put the reporter in league with the psychiatric community's convoluted idea of scientific standards, but the reporter does not provide any scientific proof to back up her claim. Rather, Connor refers to a mouthpiece of the APA to provide another bizarre opinion that "the treatments work...we have demonstrated that through robust scientific study." Hello, Earth to planet psycho-pharma. Scully's response is interesting, given that the FDA's 2004 review of antidepressant clinical trial data does not support his findings (at least in the adolescent population). The FDA is still reviewing the data to decide if adults fare any better than adolescents.

Beyond that, does it seem remotely possible that Scully, the medical director of the premier psychiatric association in the U.S., missed the FDA public health advisories drawing attention to the concerns raised about the safety and efficacy of antidepressants in the adolescent and adult population, prompting "black box" warnings? Is it possible that Scully missed the FDA's public warnings that the antidepressants used to treat these alleged mental illnesses may increase suicidal thoughts and other harmful behaviors? Is it possible that Scully missed the FDA's warning that "antidepressants may increase suicidal thoughts and actions in one out of 50 people age 18 and younger? And, finally, is it possible Scully was unaware that dozens of European nations effectively have banned the use of antidepressants in adolescents due to their concerns about safety and efficacy?

Moreover, considering that the FDA public health warnings were reported by virtually every major news organization in the U.S. and around the world, does it not seem odd that Connor's article is devoid of this information?

But what is most telling about the *Daily News* article is not what *is* written but, rather, what is *not* written. If Cruise's comments, such as "there is no such thing as a chemical imbalance," are inaccurate, why did Connor provide the APA's *opinion* about the drug treatments, rather than provide the scientific evidence disproving the actor's comments about the chemical imbalance? Wouldn't scientific proof for just one psychiatric diagnosis, such as depression, being caused by a "chemical imbalance" put Cruise in his place and end further debate?

The reason for the glaringly obvious omission is the fact that Cruise is right: There is no objective, confirmable abnormality to substantiate that a "chemical imbalance" exists in any living human brain or that a "chemical imbalance" is the cause of any psychiatric diagnosis. This also may explain why the APA's Scully did not provide the science to back up his remarks but, rather, came up with the ever so clever yet pointless "the world is flat" remark.

It's easy to understand the difficulties reporters face getting answers to these questions, as I experienced the same difficulties during my six years of reporting the issue. It was exactly these kinds of non-answers that prompted me to look into the issue deeper. And even during the writing of this book I have been unable to get a single pharmaceutical company or the FDA to respond to my inquiries. But the questions have to be asked because I do agree with the psychiatric community that the well-being of many may depend on the mental health information the public is fed.

Dr. Fred A. Baughman Jr., a pediatric neurologist and a fellow of the American Academy of Neurology and author of *The ADHD Fraud: How Psychiatry Makes "Patients" of Normal Children*, has done what most would expect of the nation's reporters—he has repeatedly requested from the most respected psycho-wizards the scientific proof to substantiate the psychiatric brain "disease" claim, including the following request to the top banana in psychiatry, Dr. Steven Sharfstein, the APA's president. Baughman's August 2005 letter to Sharfstein is representative of good science and reads (in part):

"I have discovered and described real diseases. Such discoveries are the subject of the first, single, original case report of this disease/ syndrome/abnormality or that I have discovered, described and enlarged upon existing descriptions of other real diseases as well,

but this is sufficient to make the point that for every real disease, there is just one, original case report.

I request at this time that you provide me with the citation to the first case report/validation you have for any "mental illness." Why not start with a few of psychiatry's better known, more highly publicized "diseases": OCD, ADHD, ODD, major depression, post-partum depression, bi-polar disorder, PTSD, panic disorder, conduct disorder and generalized anxiety disorder. If any of the above are real diseases, such original case reports must exist and should be readily at hand for the purpose of a prompt response."[2]

Baughman did not receive a reply to this request. In numerous other requests Baughman made, rather than receive the specific citations to the validating proof of disease, the respected neurologist was insultingly referred to textbooks.

Baughman is among many neurologists questioning the validity of the claims by the psychiatric community that the alleged mental illnesses are diseases of the brain. Yet these physicians rarely are called upon by the mainstream media to provide the factual opposing view to the psychiatric community's claims, relegating them to the editorial and commentary sections of newspapers and websites.

Dr. John M. Friedberg is another neurologist who has taken a firm stand against the fraud of psychiatric disease. The San Francisco-based neurologist felt compelled to respond to the attack against Cruise, specifically directing his comments to the remarks made by New Jersey Gov. Richard J. Codey, whose wife has publicly discussed her struggle with depression. Friedberg refers to the textbooks to back up his assertions; he writes, in part:

"The Governor of New Jersey, Richard Codey, poised to launch an ambitious first-ever statewide screening and drugging program for children with "chemical imbalances," went head on over the holiday weekend against Tom Cruise: "Tom Cruise knows as much about postpartum depression as I do about acting, and he should stick to acting and not talk about women who need help." While I sympathize with Mrs. Codey's suffering, I certainly do not agree that her experience makes her an expert or that her failed example should be forced on others. Especially children!

With regard to Attention Deficit Disorder in children, look it up. ADD isn't so much as indexed in the most authoritative textbooks of pathology. And while you're in the index of Robbins Texbook of Pathology, *check for bipolar disorder. Not there. Post partum depression, not there. And then check for schizophrenia, the mental illness of all mental illnesses, also not there.*

Pathology, which for two centuries has been the foundation of medical science, has no patience for irreproducible results. It has plenty of real diseases to document. You won't find spring fever or heartbreak either. To date, there are no provable chemical imbalances in any mental illness, at least not until brain disabling drugs and electroshock has been given and then the effects can be dramatic."[3]

Baughman and Friedberg are not isolated cases of physicians who have been outspoken critics of the psychiatric brain disease. There are numerous physicians who have stepped up to the plate to try and set the record straight. Nevertheless, regardless of the medical/scientific argument the doctors put forward, it is the psychiatric community that is hailed as the ultimate expert opinion and these brave doctors are marginalized and shunned by their peers and ignored by major news organizations. Even *The Washington Post*, one of the nation's top newspapers and famous for its Watergate investigative hounds Bob Woodward and Carl Bernstein, often fails to accurately report the facts of psychiatric diagnosing.

For example, in response to the Cruise-Lauer debacle *Washington Post* staff writer Richard Leiby wrote *"A Couch Tom Cruise Won't Jump On,"* a 600-word diatribe about the actor's delivery and his affiliation with the Church of Scientology. Rather than responsibly report the facts of Cruise's comments, Leiby wrote "Cruise looked like a man possessed—or at least in need of an Ativan..."[4]

While Leiby apparently thought the Ativan line was humorous, suggesting Cruise needed a sedative, the adverse reactions to this mind-altering drug are not funny and may include *increased aggressiveness, depression, hallucinations, depersonalization, dizziness, fatigue, disorientation, amnesia, nausea, psychomotor agitation, hostility and mental confusion* to name a few. While it is clear that Lieby intended to make light of the interview, even he would have to admit that Cruise was serious in his delivery and even called Lauer on the carpet for being "glib" in his responses.

More importantly, though, nowhere in Leiby's piece is there a discussion of whether Cruise's remarks were accurate. Rather, the writer takes the interview as an opportunity to bash the Church of Scientology, and then relies on the pharmaceutical industry-supported mental health lobby, Children and Adults With Attention Deficit/Hyperactivity Disorder (CHADD), to take up the psycho-pharma crusade in a response which has nothing to do with science but is as sarcastic as APA medical director Scully's "world is flat" remark. The best CHADD's talking head could come up with is "Since when would a celebrity have expertise in medicine? Would you go to your doctor and ask him about movie roles?" Obviously, most Americans would agree with CHADD's assessment, unless, of course, the reporter had made them aware that Cruise was accurate in his claims. Leiby failed to mention this fact and, rather than thoughtfully address the deadly serious issue, the reporter turned the interview into a farce.

There are exceptions, though, and it appears that Cruise's passionate response did in fact provide a long-needed, yet, short-lived, public debate. One month after the Cruise-Lauer interview, *Today Show* anchorwoman Katie Couric interviewed APA President Sharfstein and Harvard Medical School professor and author Dr. Joseph Glenmullen to discuss the issues Cruise had raised. The following conversation is provided in part:

Couric: But so are some painkillers, to be perfectly honest. Does that mean that painkillers shouldn't be prescribed?

Dr. Glenmullen: But—but patients should be told. They should be told when they start these drugs. Psychiatric drugs can mask the real problems. Psychiatric drugs are being overprescribed. **He's (Cruise) right when he actually says that there are no proven biochemical imbalances. Everyone's shocked by that, but it's true, and we don't want to lose sight of the very real issues that he's raised.**

Couric: Well, let me talk to Dr. Sharfstein about that. What about—he said there's no such thing as a chemical imbalance. Tell us your reaction to that.

Dr. Sharfstein: Well, that's just total nonsense. It belies the last 20 years of incredible breakthroughs in neuroscience and our understanding of how the brain works, and the fact that the medications that we use are very helpful—often very helpful."[5] (Emphasis added)

Sharfstein's comments are pure boilerplate psycho-wizard rebuttals and the APA's president does not provide specific science to support his "that's just total nonsense" statement for even one psychiatric diagnosis. Furthermore, Sharfstein does not say that a chemical imbalance exists and, because the top psycho-wizard is smart enough to know that television is all about sound bites, he knew he could get away with not directly answering the question but, instead, fire back with the incredulous non-response "that's just total nonsense."

As a side note, having read Dr. Glenmullen's books, which clearly lay out why there is no such thing as "chemical imbalance" in the living human brain (see Chapter 3), I could only wonder what was going through the Harvard doctor's mind when Sharfstein, on national television, in essence had called him a liar at worst and, at best, had insulted his intelligence.

Nevertheless, in the world of 15-second TV sound bites, Sharfstein could be comfortable in his assumption that Couric would not follow up with asking him for the specific validating scientific evidence to substantiate his response—proof that a chemical imbalance exists— and she didn't. The top shrink's response to Couric takes on a whole new meaning, though, when one recalls that this is the same Dr. Sharfstein who provided the deceptive comment in the July 11, 2005, People magazine: "We do not have a clean-cut lab test" [to determine a chemical imbalance in the brain] (see Chapter 3).

It is also Dr. Sharfstein who is quoted in the APA's official response to the Cruise-Lauer interview when in a June 27, 2005, press release he continues the psychiatric crusade (in part) "It is irresponsible for Mr. Cruise to use his movie publicity tour to promote his own ideological views and deter people with mental illness from getting the care they need. It is unfortunate that in the face of this remarkable scientific and clinical progress that a small number of individuals and groups persist in questioning its legitimacy."[6]

This is beautiful. Nowhere in the entire APA press release does the top shrink state that Cruise is incorrect in his comments but, rather, Sharfstein's response is focused on the audacity of the Hollywood superstar to so much as even question the legitimacy of psychiatric diagnosing, that Cruise's accurate comments—which are the truth—are somehow hurting people. It apparently never occurred to the APA president that people like Cruise and others "persist" in questioning the legitimacy of psychiatric diagnosing because there is no objective, confirmable science to support a single psychiatric mental illness being caused by an abnormality of the brain. But Sharfstein apparently comes from the school of "if psychiatry says it enough it becomes fact" (IPSIEIBF).

As a follow up to his *Today Show* appearance Sharfstein, apparently pleased with his TV debut with Couric, two weeks later published in *Psychiatric News* (the trade magazine of the psychiatric community) a piece titled "My 15 Minutes of Fame" in which he reminisces about his plan of attack for the *Today Show* interview and explains "most importantly, we can get the word out that psychiatric illness is real disease..."[7] (IPSIEIBF) Ugh!

Even when broadcast journalism seems to get it right, at least making a show of asking the important questions; it appears this kind of responsible in-depth interviewing is temporary. Six months after the *Today Show* interview with Drs. Sharfstein and Glenmullen, Couric conducts another interview that leaves one wondering if the darling of morning television is deliberately trying to minimize the issue. During a December 2005 interview on NBC's *Dateline* program with investigative broadcast journalist Mike Wallace, Couric appears to be clueless on the psychiatric drugging issue and, again, the viewing public is left with opinions rather than accurate information (in part):

Couric: How do you feel about Tom Cruise's assertion that...

Wallace: Scientology and so forth is going to help you and the e-meter and all that?

Couric: Well, that antidepressants aren't good, that there's no use for them.

Wallace: I think he doesn't know what he's talking about. He doesn't know what he's talking about.[8]

Did Couric forget what was said in her earlier interview—there is no such thing as a chemical imbalance? Apparently so, and rather than follow a line of questioning that deals in specifics about the alleged chemical imbalance, or perhaps the now well-known dangers associated with antidepressant use in an unknown number of the population, something along the lines of "Mike, the FDA this year issued public health advisories raising concerns about the safety and efficacy of antidepressants, what do you think about that?" Couric throws the *60 Minutes* star and admitted long-time user of mind-altering drugs a softball question about whether he *thinks* antidepressants are good! What did Couric expect Wallace would say? "No, Katie, Tom Cruise is right. I hate antidepressants, they don't work?" This line of questioning can only be described as fluff and a disservice not only to Cruise but also the television-viewing public. Cruise is correct in his comments that psychiatric mental disorders are not brain-based diseases and, yet, it is the icon of investigative journalism, Mike Wallace, apparently based on his personal use of antidepressants, who decides Cruise knows not of what he speaks.

But this raises another interesting aspect of the Cruise-Lauer interview: It is the media that has appointed itself planet psycho-pharma referee, arbitrarily deciding which celebrity is right and which is wrong. Despite the fact that Cruise's remarks were accurate, he nevertheless was portrayed in the media as a crazed Scientologist. On the other hand, Brooke Shields, who openly discusses her use of antidepressants as treatment for her experience with depression after delivering her first child, was embraced by the media as a kind of modern day Joan of Arc. Shields provides no scientific evidence—nothing in the way of objective, confirmable proof—that her alleged "post-partum" depression is a real disease or that the mind-altering drugs she took as treatment specifically target the alleged mental abnormality and, yet, she is portrayed by the media as the pathetic wounded starlet.

Apparently, how celebrity credibility is established on the issue of psychiatric diagnosing depends on whether the celebrity has a personal history with alleged mental illnesses and mind-altering drug use. The media's ground rules appear to be something along the lines of "if you've been diagnosed mentally ill and used mind-altering drugs but have no science to back up your claims, we support you, but if you've never taken mind-altering drugs and your information is accurate, you're crazed."

Peter Breggin M.D., internationally known psychiatrist, author of more than a dozen books, including *Talking Back to Prozac*, *Toxic Psychiatry* and *Talking Back to Ritalin*, and ever the man of logic and reason, eloquently explained his take on the Cruise-Lauer interview (in part):

"Tom cruise did the unthinkable on TV. Actually, he did several "unthinkables" in a filmed interview with NBC's Matt Lauer for the Today Show. *First, Tom pointed out that Matt Lauer actually was very "glib" (shallow) and didn't know what he was talking about. He also urged Matt to be "more responsible" and to learn something about psychiatry before touting it. For a star to do this to a media personality was unthinkable. Since nearly all of them are shallow, this was a threat of potentially epidemic proportions. Suppose other guests began pointing out that media hosts don't know what they are talking about and are shallow?*

Why was the media both drawn into the story and shocked by it? It was too good a story to simply ignore. "Tom Cruise Gone Wild!" was the theme. It should have been "Tom Cruise Gets Serious." The media would have liked to attack Tom on the grounds that he's a Scientologist. Scientologists seem to share a number of views about psychiatry with me, including everything Tom said.

In fact, I'd go further. Modern biological psychiatry is a materialistic religion masquerading as science. How can I say that my profession of psychiatry is a materialistic religion? Because modern psychiatry makes believe that psychological and spiritual problems, such as anxiety and depression, are caused by mechanical failures in the physical brain, and because psychiatry then attempts to correct these psychological and spiritual problems with physical interventions such as drugs and electroshock."[9]

The above doctors who came out in support of Cruise, substantiating his comments about psychiatric diagnosing, are just a sample of a very long list, yet there are no pithy headlines in major newspapers or on TV news shows giving the actor his due and correcting the inaccurate information. The public's perception of Cruise unfairly remains that of the crazed Scientologist (whatever that is) making wild, unsubstantiated claims and America moseys along in an altered state of psychiatric reality. This is no accident. There is much at stake for the powerful psycho-pharma industry, and tens of billions of dollars are riding on continuing the illusion that Americans suffer from the alleged mental *diseases*.

A January 2005 study conducted by Brandeis University reports that prescription psychotropic (mind-altering) drug use among teenagers "skyrocketed 250 percent between 1994 and 2001."[10] The study further reveals that "by 2001, one in every ten of all office visits by teenage boys led to a prescription for a psychotropic drug." And the study's authors also report that "a diagnosis of ADHD was given in about one-third of office visits during the period, and between 14 and 26 percent of visits in which psychotropic medications were prescribed did not have an associated mental health diagnosis."

This is amazing. The Brandeis data reveals that mind-altering drugs are doled out to the oblivious public without even so much as a suggestion of a mental illness diagnosis. In other words, the use of psychiatric mind-altering drugs has become so commonplace, so accepted by the public that the guise of being labeled mentally ill isn't even necessary to get them. This, of course, is great news for the pharmaceutical companies but does not bode well for the psychiatric profession, as it more or less eliminates or, at the very least, minimizes whatever specialty the physicians claimed to possess. Nor does it bode well for the future of this great nation when an ever-increasing number of the population apparently is in need of having their minds chemically altered on a daily basis just to function "normally."

The authors of the study conclude that there are a number of reasons for the enormous increase in mind-altering drug use, including "greater acceptance among physicians and the public of psychotropic drugs, the advent of new medications with fewer side effects, increased screening for mental disorders and patient demand for such drugs." Is it possible that the public has "greater acceptance" of psychiatric mind-altering drugs because America's press corps has failed to accurately cover the issue of psychiatric diagnosing? In other words, rather than continue to regurgitate the lie of the psycho-pharma brain disease, what would the nation's mind-altering drug use be had the press repeatedly reported that there is no science to support even a single psychiatric mental illness is caused by an objective confirmable abnormality in the brain? A good clue can be found in the following news article which demonstrates that if the American people are given *all* the information, they will act accordingly.

In October 2005 *The Washington Post* ran a front-page, above-the-fold article by staff writer Shankar Vedantam titled *"Psychiatric Drugs' Use Drops for Children."*[11] Vedantam provides an excellent report about the nearly 20 percent drop in pediatric use of mind-altering drugs that occurred after the FDA issued public health warnings about antidepressants being no more effective than sugar pills in a majority of clinical trials, and that the mind-altering drugs may increase suicidal behavior. Vedantam covers the issue like a seasoned reporter, providing comments about the safety and efficacy of the antidepressants in question from those who advocate the virtues of the mind-altering drugs to those opposed and why.

While the *Post* reporter provided good insight into the ongoing debate about the benefits and risks of mind-altering drugs, like so many reporters covering the psycho/pharma issue, nowhere in the article is mention made about the legitimacy of the psychiatric diagnosing. Instead, by leaving out any discussion by experts questioning the legitimacy of the psychiatric diagnosis, which leads to the prescribing of the mind-altering drugs, the lengthy news piece by default provides credence to the pseudoscience of subjective psychiatric diagnosing. Once again it is the mind-altering drugs that take the limelight, and the legitimacy of the alleged mental illnesses is not even a consideration. And, although credit is due to the *Post* for its comprehensive coverage of the psycho-pharma debate, in its apparent eagerness to report recent developments, the paper sometimes gets the proverbial cart before the horse.

A Jan. 1, 2006, *Post* front-page article by Ron Stein and Marc Kaufman headlined *"Depression Drugs Safe, Beneficial, Studies Say: Suicide Risk Rejected, But Critics Question Validity of Findings,"* covers in some detail the results of two taxpayer-funded studies that report to negate the FDA's earlier conclusions about the potentially deadly risks associated with antidepressant use, which moved the FDA to request of the pharmaceutical companies to place "black box" warnings on the psychiatric mind-altering drugs.

The lead paragraph of the Stein-Kaufman article is indicative of the kind of psychiatric misinformation that permeates the press: "Antidepressants, such as Prozac and similar drugs, help many patients overcome their often disabling psychiatric *disease* and do not increase the risk for suicide in adults, according to two large studies being published today that counter recent concerns about the popular medications"[12] (italics mine). Is it any wonder that prescription psychiatric drug use increases exponentially year after year? The *Post*, known for its extraordinary investigative reporters, says psychiatric mental disorders are *diseases,* so they must be!

Whether or not an alleged mental disorder is a disease is no small matter, especially when one considers that the Stein-Kaufman article is reporting that the mind-altering antidepressants actually treat the alleged diseases. Since there is no proof of an objective, confirmable abnormality of the brain for any psychiatric diagnosis, many may wonder just what are the psychiatric drugs treating? There is no known brain abnormality for depression, OCD, postpartum depression, anxiety or any of the other psychiatric diagnoses. In fact, in the case of psychiatric drugs, pharmaceutical-company sponsored clinical trials depend on the participant's verbal response to questions about their behavior to determine whether the drug is effective, not objective scientific pathological proof that a brain abnormality even exists—subsequently making it impossible to know if the phantom abnormality has been eliminated or even measurably minimized.

Despite the reporters' initial misinformation, the article spells out in detail the results of the two NIMH-funded studies that reviewed health insurance data and also analysis of clinical practice patient information. The results of the two studies showed no increased risk of suicide with the newer antidepressants. However, just nine days later, Dr. Robert Temple, the medical policy director of the FDA's Center for Drug Evaluation and Research, is quoted in the FDA "Pink Sheet" stating: "The new study bears only a tangential relationship at best to the previous information." Temple further explained, "The previous analysis that led to the "black box" [warning] was a comparison between drugs and placebo in people who are depressed, and it compared the likelihood of suicidality in the drug-treated and placebo-treated patients. The new study doesn't have an untreated group. They have no information at all about what would have happened to those people had they not been treated. It simply sheds no light at all on the particular point raised in the labeling or the analysis of those trials."[13]

In other words, the lead drug approver at the FDA sees no benefit from the largely hyped studies because neither study compares treated patients against untreated patients, leaving the question, according to Temple, "what would have happened to those people had they not been treated," unanswered. In short, the studies do not take into consideration how many of the patients would have gotten "better" without drug treatment—the studies do not compare treated patients against untreated nor is there a comparison of the benefit of one drug treatment against another.

Given the FDA's take on the studies, the quote provided in the Stein-Kaufman article from Darrel A. Regier, the director of research for the APA, seems laughable: *"What the FDA initiated was in some ways a natural experiment...this is the kind of rigorous scientific information the FDA should consider in evaluating its decisions."* It is not surprising that the premier psychiatric organization would find that the flawed studies provide scientifically rigorous information, as these are the same deep thinkers that push the fraud of psychiatric brain disease.

Although the *Post* reporters devoted three sentences in the article to the contrarian's side, or "critics" view, of the studies, the bulk of the 900-word news article is devoted to the results of the now admittedly flawed studies. And, at the time of this writing, the *Post* has not run a follow-up front-page article exposing the serious flaws of the studies; the paper's front-page headline, "Depression

Drugs Safe, Beneficial, Studies Say," is what its reading public is left with.

Five days after the above article was published by the *Post*, the paper ran another article under its "Findings" section, which contains brief news accounts by various media outlets of recent scientific discoveries. The five-paragraph news item titled *"Researchers Link a Protein to Depression,"* is another good example of why America remains clueless about the fraud of psychiatric diagnosing. For example, the unauthored article states: "Scientists have discovered a protein that *seems* to play a crucial role in developing depression, a finding that *may* lead to new treatments for the often debilitating illness—and fundamental understanding of why it strikes."[14] (italics mine)

So the first paragraph tells the reader many things, including that the hopeful discovery is not certain but may lead to why depression strikes. In other words, the discovery may reveal the cause of depression. So far, so good, but it gets more interesting. The second paragraph explains: "Although problems with the mood-regulating brain chemical serotonin have long been linked to depression, scientists do not know what causes the **disease** that afflicts some 18 million Americans—or exactly what serotonin's role is."[15] (Emphasis added) Ha, ha, ha, this is brilliant!

The unknown author not only out-and-out states that the scientific community is clueless about the cause of depression but, apparently disregarding the demonstrative statement, decides to call depression a *disease* anyway. UGH! If science has not discovered an objective, confirmable abnormality in the brain that is depression, how can science possibly know depression is a disease? Furthermore, the author of the article also admits that science does not know "exactly what serotonin's role is." Really, what happened to the chemical imbalance, which these mind-altering drugs are alleged to treat? Of course, as has been well-established in several chapters of this book, the FDA and pharmaceutical companies openly admit that the way in which the mind-altering drugs "work" for the stated alleged mental illnesses, is a mystery. The scientific community cannot say with certainty what serotonin's role is in the treatment of any psychiatric mental illness. Finally, though, after briefly explaining how the protein "appears" to regulate brain cells, the reporter ends the article with another demonstrative yet unproven statement that "most depression drugs used today work by making more serotonin available to brain cells."

Although it is believed, thought and suggested that increasing serotonin levels in the brain treats depression, there is no objective, confirmable proof that the drugs treat any known depression center. Even the pharmaceutical companies that manufacture the mind-altering drugs at least have the integrity to qualify the way or method in which the companies' drugs allegedly work in the treatment of the alleged mental illness by adding the caveats "may," "thought" "believes" and "suggests." Furthermore, with the FDA's 2004 review of antidepressant clinical trial data showing that the sugar pill (placebo) was as effective as the antidepressant "treatment" in a majority of the drugs reviewed, the jury still is out on whether the mind-altering drugs "treat" anything. What is certain is that psychiatric mind-altering drugs—antidepressants—disrupt the naturally occurring chemicals in the brain. Anything more specific, regardless of the number of years science has been conducting research on brain chemicals, is pure speculation.

Generally, the mainstream media, whether deliberately or through ignorance, has missed the importance of covering the facts of the psycho-pharma debate. Repeatedly, alleged mental illnesses are inaccurately referred to as disease, and the debate surrounding the legitimacy of psychiatric diagnosing is not so much as even mentioned. Subsequently, the American public is forced to accept as truth blatant inaccuracies, relegating the still-curious to turn to alternative news sources such as the Internet, to get a more complete view not provided by the psycho-pharma establishment (see Appendix B). But even this medium is limited, especially in light of the large number of the population, including the elderly and very young, who may be unable to tap into the information superhighway.

There are a handful of reporters, though, who regularly cover the issue with the kind of in-depth investigative curiosity that many would expect for an issue that increasingly is becoming, and should be addressed as, one of public safety. New York-based freelance

179

medical journalist Jeanne Lenzer is one such reporter, and often is published in the *British Medical Journal* (*BMJ*). Through dogged pursuit, Lenzer has consistently held the feet of the scientific community and the pharmaceutical industry to the fire. Lenzer's coverage of the psycho-pharma industry is some of the best in journalism today, but is by no means the only example.

The Washington Times—the "other" newspaper in Washington, D.C.—consistently provides responsible coverage of the psycho-pharma debate, including a July 7, 2005, dead-on commentary by Keith Hoeller titled "War of Two Religious Worldviews," which nailed the facts of the Cruise-Lauer interview. Hoeller writes (in part):

"All his statements went against the dominant ideology, as espoused by "Today" host Matt Lauer. To get his point across, Mr. Cruise had to interrupt Mr. Lauer, who kept framing the questions within the framework of psychiatry.

After his expression of a heretical view, the mental health movement's high priests promptly went into action. The American Psychiatric Association and the National Alliance for the Mentally Ill, both heavily funded by drug companies, assured the public Mr. Cruise was wrong and the mentally ill need and benefit from their daily psychiatric drugs.

However, neither the APA, nor NAMI, nor Miss [Brooke] Shields offered any credible scientific evidence to support their claims that depressed people have a bona fide chemical imbalance that is cured by antidepressant drugs. For in fact psychiatrists have yet to conclusively prove any mental illness is caused by a chemical imbalance of any kind."[16]

The problem for most reporters, of course, is that the accuracy of reporting on the psycho-pharma debate largely depends on information provided by the talking heads of the psychiatric community, and specifically the APA. As has been well-established, the premier psychiatric association routinely spouts the brain disease line and rarely, if ever, is forced to prove its claims. In fact, as in the case of the Cruise-Lauer interview, for example, the standard operating procedure of the psychiatric community is to personally attack the messenger rather than responsibly, through scientific proof, respond to the message. The powerful APA, backed by the financial muscle of the pharmaceutical companies, *BELIEVES* so deeply in the psychiatric brain disease theory that anyone who dares question the claim, with the assistance of mainstream media, is reduced to public humiliation. The APA and psychiatric community has so often said mental illnesses are diseases of the brain that it permeates the national psyche—and the claim couldn't be further from the truth. And, yet, it is the nation's press corps that fails to accurately inform the American people each and every time the medical/psychiatric community is allowed to regurgitate as fact the psychiatric brain disease line.

In searching the Internet for news articles about the psycho-pharma debate I ran across an interesting piece run in *The Washingtonian* magazine titled "Stop the Presses! Pass the Prozac!" which *Post* White House reporter Dana Milbank is reported to have told an audience at Yale, his alma mater, that "40 percent of the *Post* reporters are on antidepressants." In the brief *Washingtonian* piece, when questioned Milbank clarified his comments saying "I wasn't meaning to limit that to my colleagues. Industrywide, it's quite common. I include *The Washingtonian*."[17]

While it is anyone's guess if Milbank's data is correct, if it is even close, it may explain the media's pro-psycho-pharma stand and why today it very much appears the psycho-pharma debate truly is a case of the blind leading the blind. But, Americans are beginning to understand the adverse reactions to the popular mind-altering drugs, which may eventually lead to better coverage of the psychiatric diagnosing debate. And, in the wake of the FDA warnings about antidepressants and other prescription drugs, the People have begun to fight back, filing an ever-increasing number of personal injury and wrongful death lawsuits against the pharmaceutical industry. Not surprisingly, the lawsuits focus on the harm caused by the mind-altering drugs, while the psychiatric community escapes scrutiny.

Kelly Patricia O'Meara

[1] Tracy Connor, *The New York Daily News*, "Tom a pill on TV," June 24, 2005

[2] Fred A. Baughman, Jr., M.D., "Letter to APA President Steven Sharfstein," August 2005

[3] John M. Friedberg, M.D., "Pharmaceutical Fundamentalism: A Neurologist Speaks Out On Chemical Imbalances," San Francisco, *Indymedia*, July 2005.

[4] Richard Leiby, "A Couch Tom Cruise Won't Jump On: Actor Lambastes Psychiatry on 'Today,'" *The Washington Post*, June 25, 2005

[5] Katie Couric, Dr. Steven Sharfstein and Dr. Joseph Glenmullen, Today Show Interview Transcript, June 27, 2005.

[6] Steven S. Sharfstein, M.D., "APA Responds to Tom Cruise's Today Show Interview," APA Press Release, June 27, 2005.

[7] Steven S. Sharfstein, M.D., "My 15 Minutes of Fame," *Psychiatric News*, August 5, 2005.

[8] Katie Couric, "Mike Wallace, Man of the Hour," Dateline Interview, December 9, 2005

[9] Peter R. Breggin, M.D., "Dr. Peter Breggin: Thanks Tom Cruise," HuffingtonPost. com, July 17, 2005.

[10] Brandeis University "Psychotropic Drug Prescriptions for Teens Surge 250 Percent Over Seven Years," *Journal Psychiatric Services*, January 3, 2006.

[11] Shankar Vedantam, "Psychiatric Drugs' Use Drops for Children," *The Washington Post*, October 8, 2005.

[12] Ron Stein and Marc Kaufman, "Depression Drugs Safe, Beneficial, Studies Say: Suicide Risk Rejected, But Critics Question Validity of Findings," *The Washington Post*, January 1, 2006.

[13] "FDA Stance on Antidepressant Warnings Unchanged By NIMH Suicide Findings," Pink Sheet, January 9, 2006. Volume 68, Number 002, pg-16.

[14] "Researchers Link A Protein to Depression," *The Washington Post*, January 6, 2006.

[15] Ibid.

[16] Keith Hoeller, "War of Two Religious Worldviews," *The Washington Times*, July 7, 2005.

[17] Chuck Conconi, "Stop the Presses! Pass the Prozac," Capital Comment, *Washingtonian Magazine*, May 2003

Chapter Nine

Planet Psycho-Pharma on Trial

If ever there was any doubt about where the FDA's loyalties lie, the answer to that question was delivered in the agency's "we're-looking-out-for-your-best-interest" voice via a Jan. 18, 2005, press release titled "FDA Announces New Prescription Drug Information Format to Improve Patient Safety."

The federal drug approval agency was trumpeting its long-awaited revisions—the first in 25 years—to the format of prescription drug package inserts, which the agency claims will "provide the most up-to-date information in an easy-to-read format that draws physician and patient attention to the most important pieces of drug information before a product is prescribed."[1] There's a new concept: providing the public drug package inserts that actually can be understood by someone who doesn't hold a Ph.D. in chemistry.

On the surface the revisions seem like good news, right? Yes and no. It appears that in its effort to "improve the packaging inserts" the FDA also decided to delve into legaldom's tort law, building in for its good friends at Planet psycho-pharma a gilded exit door to escape an ever-increasing number of lawsuits.

The FDA's smooth move was not missed by the media, and according to a Jan. 14, 2005, article in *The Wall Street Journal* (*WSJ*), the FDA "is preparing to declare that federally approved medication labels pre-empt state law."[2] And, in a Jan. 19, 2006, article in *The Washington Post*, the FDA's deputy commissioner for medical and scientific affairs, Scott Gottlieb, explained the federal pre-emption policy saying, "We think that if your company complies with the FDA processes, if you bring forward the benefits and risks of your drug and let your information be judged through a process with highly trained scientists, you should not be second-guessed by state courts that don't have the same scientific knowledge."[3] Even to the untrained ear, one would have to admit the FDA official's comments are eerily similar to those of the American Psychiatric Association (APA) about those people who have the audacity to "persist" in questioning the legitimacy of psychiatric diagnosing.

In essence, though, what the FDA has proposed is that if the drug approval agency gives its seal of approval to a new drug, with all the bells and whistles about adverse reactions attached to the labels and inserts, then the pharmaceutical companies should be protected from personal injury and wrongful death lawsuits filed in state courts due to their prescription drugs and all liability lawsuits should be heard in federal court (the federal pre-emption standard). It is unclear how the FDA could even suggest such a policy in light of the recent Vioxx debacle, but beyond that there are a few other huge problems with the suggested policy decision, the least of which is made crystal clear in the case of the 2004 "black box" warnings placed on all antidepressants.

Recall that it was the same "highly trained scientists" at the FDA who for more than a decade refused to place warnings on antidepressants about increased risks of suicide and other harmful behaviors in patients taking the drugs, despite the fact that tens of thousands of adverse reactions, including suicide and attempted suicide, were reported to the agency's adverse event reporting system (AERS). This also is the same group of deep thinkers who, despite being forced by the public to hold hearings in 1991 about the new class of antidepressants because of reports of an ever-increasing number of suicides and other harmful behaviors, decided the data being reviewed were inconclusive and therefore there was no need to warn the public. The public is just supposed to forget that half of the 1991 FDA committee members who voted against adding additional warnings to the antidepressants had conflicts of interests due to their professional and financial ties with the pharmaceutical companies that manufactured the antidepressants being reviewed. Due to these conflicts of interest, it only took the "highly trained scientists" at the FDA 13 years to act in the best interest of the American public.

And many would argue that the federal drug approval agency only acted in 2004 because the British had a year earlier forced its hand, effectively banning the use of antidepressants in the adolescent population in Great Britain. And, not to beat a dead horse, why should the American people trust the psycho-wizards at the FDA when it is these same "highly trained scientists" who apparently are incapable of providing the public with the detailed information about when the agency received the "missing" Eli Lilly data.

This is no small issue when one considers that if the FDA had received the admittedly damning Prozac information prior to the drug's U.S. approval, then the public certainly would have to wonder just whose interests were being served by the federal drug approval agency. Ultimately, though, there are several specific reasons why Americans may find the FDA's new policy recommendations, effectively stripping away the right to bring legal action against the pharmaceutical companies in state court, unworthy of the public's confidence or support.

While there have been dozens of books written about the "wonder" drug Prozac, the first SSRI marketed in the U.S., there is one author who has done for understanding the dangers of Prozac and other antidepressants what the late Carl Sagan did for understanding the cosmos. In his 1994 book, *Talking Back to Prozac: What Doctors Aren't Telling You About Today's Most Controversial Drug*, Peter Breggin M.D. explains the unique scientific methods that are utilized by pharmaceutical companies—in this instance, Eli Lilly and Co.—in order to get FDA approval for new drugs. In Chapter 3 of *Talking Back to Prozac*, Breggin explains the questionable clinical trial data that was provided to the FDA listing several specific points about the methods utilized by Lilly in order to prove the safety and efficacy of its new psychiatric mind-altering drug. For instance, Breggin points out that the FDA allowed "a very questionable but commonly used technique in the drugs studies: placebo washout."[4] In a nutshell, "placebo washout" consists of all patients in a clinical trial all starting out on a placebo (sugar pill). The patients who improve on the placebo are dropped from the clinical trials and the study begins anew with the remaining patients. The placebo washout, says Breggin, "purposely produces an unnatural pool of patients. It is unscientific."[5]

Breggin further reports that "the Prozac studies, as designed by Lilly, excluded all patients with serious tendencies toward suicide… and hospitalized psychiatric patients were also excluded from nearly all of the studies, including every one that was used to approve the drug."[6] Adding to the list of people not represented in the clinical trials of Prozac are children and the elderly—a particularly important point given that the drug has been prescribed to the elderly, while the "off-label" prescribing of the drug to children is well-documented by the 2004 FDA hearings, which resulted in "black box" warnings for all antidepressants.

Another point of contention, according to Breggin, is the totals of patients reportedly participating in the clinical trials and actually taking the drug. Breggin reveals an interesting progression of funny patient numbers. "In a 'Dear Doctor' letter written by Eli Lilly to American physicians to counteract concerns that Prozac could increase suicidality, the letter states, 'More than 11,000 individuals participated in clinical trials for Prozac, including over 6,000 treated with Prozac.'" Breggin points out that the "Dear Doctor" letter reflects that it is "over 6,000" who actually took Prozac, not 11,000. Furthermore, Breggin points to the drug label reprinted in the *Physicians' Desk Reference* (*PDR*) that there were "5,600" who actually took the drug during clinical trials. However, in an effort to get a better understanding of those patients who actually took Prozac during pre-marketing studies, Breggin, through the Freedom of Information Act, "went through each of these seventeen studies, one by one, to add up the number of Prozac patients who actually completed the four-, five-, or six-week trials used as the basis for FDA approval. The grand total turned out to be a meager 286 patients."[7]

But Breggin's conclusion on the exact numbers of patients in clinical trials who actually took the drug is truly frightening when one considers the recent warnings on antidepressants. The psychiatrist reports "only 63 patients were on fluoxetine for a period of more than two years before completion of the pre-marketing studies and the FDA approval of Prozac. In effect, anyone now taking Prozac for more than a few weeks is part of a giant ongoing experiment on its longer-term effects."[8]

Another point is well made by Breggin when one considers the FDA's recent suggested policy changes, which effectively would exempt pharmaceutical companies from litigation in state courts. "According to the FDA approval process, it doesn't matter how many times a drug *fails* to prove useful in its clinical trials. Innumerable scientific studies can show the drug to be ineffective, but as long as two or more show statistical superiority over placebo, the drug can win approval."[9] Through painstaking efforts, Breggin analyzed the numerous volumes of data submitted to the FDA for approval of Eli Lilly's Prozac and came to this conclusion: "In its 'Summary of Basis of Approval,' dated October 1988, the FDA states that fourteen protocols involving controlled studies were submitted by Lilly. Four compared Prozac to placebo, and of these, three were used by the FDA as evidence of some beneficial effect. One showed none at all. Of the remaining ten studies, eight showed Prozac to have no positive effect. Overall, there were more negative efforts than positive, but this made no difference in the approval process. In six out of the seven studies where it was included, imipramine (Tofranil), a very old drug, did better than Prozac. That, too, made no difference in the approval process."[10]

And to add insult to injury, the "missing" Lilly internal documents, which apparently reveal the company's prior knowledge of suicidality associated with the drug, were not even an issue when Breggin published *Talking Back to Prozac*. Given the number of studies that showed there was no benefit to be gained by taking Prozac and the drug still was approved, it's questionable whether the "missing" documents would have had any impact on the FDA's decision, which is supposed to ensure that the drug is safe *and* effective. But it is precisely these reasons that the drug agency's apparent desire to protect the pharmaceutical companies from lawsuits seems at the very least misguided.

The "Forsyth lawsuit" is an exceptionally pertinent example of why the FDA's suggested "get-out-of-jail-free" card serves only the interests of the pharmaceutical companies. In 1993, William Forsyth was suffering panic attacks and was prescribed Prozac as treatment. But the 63-year-old felt worse and checked into a hospital where the Prozac was continued. Eleven days after beginning Prozac "treatment," Forsyth returned home and stabbed his wife multiple times with a kitchen knife, then killed himself with the same knife.

Two of the Forsyth children sued Eli Lilly, blaming Prozac for their father's uncharacteristic actions. Only two of the hundreds of lawsuits brought against Eli Lilly by families claiming the drug had led to suicidal and other violent behaviors have ended in court verdicts. In the Forsyth case, Lilly argued that "there is absolutely no medically sound evidence of an association between any antidepressant medicine, including Prozac, and the induction of suicidal ideation or violence."[11]

Lilly's above testimony is interesting on a number of levels. First, there is no medically sound evidence that panic attacks are an abnormality—a disease—of the brain, the apparent reason that Forsyth was treated with Prozac. Furthermore, there is no objective, confirmable proof that Prozac specifically treats any psychiatric diagnosis, and the FDA makes this clear in its explanation of how Prozac works: "The antidepressant, antiobsessive-compulsive, and antibulimic actions of fluoxetine (Prozac) are presumed to be linked to its inhibition of CNS neuronal uptake of serotonin." The FDA "*presumes*" Prozac works a certain way; it does not know with any scientific certainty. Additionally, Eli Lilly's explanation of how its drug works is equally mystifying: "Depression is not fully understood, but a growing amount of evidence supports the view that people with depression have an imbalance of the brain's neurotransmitters, the chemicals that allow nerve cells in the brain to communicate with each other. Prozac may help correct this imbalance by increasing the brain's own supply of serotonin."[12] Again, given that there is no known method to test for the alleged chemical imbalance, how does any scientist, doctor or pharmaceutical company know an imbalance of naturally occurring chemicals exists in an individual living brain?

The Lilly testimony becomes pointless when one considers the FDA's 2004 conclusions about antidepressants: Suicidality in Pediatric and Adult Patients, "all patients being treated with any type of antidepressant should be observed closely for clinical worsening and suicidality especially during the first few months of therapy and when the dose is modified." The FDA included Prozac among the antidepressants listed for "black box" warnings. William Forsyth had only been on Prozac 11 days.

The FDA analysis was not available at the time of the 1999 Forsyth verdict, but another piece of interesting information was available but not provided to the Forsyth attorneys. It was due to this information that Houston-based Andy Vickory, the Forsyths' trial attorney, appealed the 1999 verdict in favor of Eli Lilly. Despite Lilly's long-held stand that there is no association between Prozac and suicidal/violent behavior, in 1998 the company paid $20 million to two doctors, with the promise of tens of millions of dollars more, for a new antidepressant patent derived from Prozac, yet concocted in such a way to decrease the adverse effects of the drug. The new drug patent reportedly decreased many of the known adverse effects, including "intense, violent, suicidal thoughts and self-mutilation." The patent language directly contradicts Lilly's assertions about the safety of Prozac, and the Forsyth family filed an appeal based on Lilly's failure to disclose the new patent information during the trial. The Forsyth case was settled before the appeals court ruled.

The pharmaceutical giant apparently forgot to mention that the new patent for which it was paying big bucks alludes to the very thing it was denying in the Forsyth case. Of course this is the big question surrounding Eli Lilly's reported commitment to providing families and doctors all the information they need, leaving one to wonder what else the company has forgotten to mention about the possible adverse effects of Prozac. But, hey, the FDA approved the drug as safe and effective. These are the same numbskulls—excuse me, "highly trained scientists"—who expect the American people to believe its drug approval decisions are beyond reproach and that they shouldn't be second-guessed? Toto, I don't think we're in Kansas anymore!

Tens of millions of Americans, including young children, have popped Prozac and other antidepressants for years on end as if it were baby aspirin, and it only took the federal drug agency 13 years to figure out that Prozac, along with all the other antidepressants on the market, may increase the risk of suicide and other harmful behaviors. But the larger question for Americans to ask is: whose mother, father, sister, brother or child is the acceptable risk, the apparent standard for allowing a drug on the market.

Given that the FDA has finally been forced to belly up to the bar about the dangers associated with antidepressants, is it any wonder that the federal drug agency finds it necessary to protect the pharmaceutical companies from lawsuits. It isn't as if suing pharmaceutical companies is new, but consider that with the new antidepressant "black box" warnings, it may have dawned on the pharmaceutical giants that there is an ever-increasing possibility that millions of Americans may begin to wonder about the tragic outcomes of loved ones who had a history of being treated with the mind-altering drugs. In fact, the ongoing lawsuits against Merck and Co. are a pretty good indication of what the pharmaceutical companies may expect should the tens of millions of antidepressant users seek relief through litigation.

Vioxx, a treatment for pain and inflammation manufactured by Merck, was approved by the FDA in 1999 and, by the time it was voluntarily pulled from the market in September 2004; at least 20 million Americans had taken the drug. Nearly 10,000 Americans have filed suit against the company claiming that early into the marketing of Vioxx the company was aware of data showing a twofold increase of heart attack and other cardiovascular risks. Although Merck has set aside $1 billion to cover the Vioxx litigation costs, many experts believe the damages could run into the tens of billions of dollars. This monetary set aside by Merck is a drop in the financial bucket compared to the revenue generated by Vioxx during its five-year run, with annual sales estimated at $2.5 billion.

In August 2004 the FDA conducted its own study that revealed the use of Vioxx was associated with thousands of heart attacks or sudden cardiac deaths. What many Americans may wonder is why the drug was approved by the FDA in the first place. Testimony provided in February 2005 by Gurkirpal Singh M.D., adjunct clinical professor of medicine in the Department of Medicine, Division of Gastroenterology and Hepatology at Stanford University School of Medicine, before the House Energy and Commerce subcommittee on Health, provides interesting insight into the drug approval process at the FDA (in part):

"In the current system of drug approval, trials designed to assess the safety of a drug are often performed after its approval—the so-called post-marketing studies. But these are rarely completed. A drug is considered 'safe' unless proven otherwise. While this system brings rapid drug approvals, it does raise the rare possibility of sometimes causing serious harm from side effects not discovered in clinical trials."[13] Dr. Singh further explained to the subcommittee, "The first principle of medicine is *primum, non nocere*—first, do no harm. It is extremely important that clinical trial data be carefully studied and if there is any indication—even a small one—that there is a possible risk of serious harm, the approval of the drug should be deferred until appropriate, large-scale data is collected."[14] In the case of Vioxx, Dr. Singh explains that the FDA was aware of early warning signs about adverse cardiovascular events associated with the drug: "In a careful review of Merck's new drug application for Vioxx, Dr. Villalba noticed that "thromboembolic events [such as heart attack and stroke] are more frequent in patients receiving Vioxx than placebo."[15] In fact, Dr. Singh explains that based on the data provided by Merck, there was a "threefold increase in the risk [of a cardiovascular event]."

Despite this early knowledge by the FDA of serious adverse events Vioxx, nevertheless, was approved, and Dr. Singh reports "there was certainly no emergent need to approve Vioxx without further studies if there were lingering safety concerns. Remember, *primum non noncere*—first, do no harm. Instead, the drug was approved by the FDA in a priority review within six months, with no discussion on the heart attack trade-off. Four years before the withdrawal of Vioxx, the FDA had "ongoing cardiovascular safety concerns surrounding Vioxx," concerns that had started before the drug was approved. Yet, the sponsor [Merck] would not do definitive studies to address these safety concerns."[16]

It appears that the FDA was aware of the concerns regarding the safety of Vioxx but decided to approve the drug anyway. Yes, it is a benefit-versus-risk world and it apparently is just unfortunate for the families of those tens of thousands who may have been harmed or even died due to adverse reactions to the drug. But this drug approval scenario is played out repeatedly by the "highly trained scientists" at the FDA who now think that its decisions should not be second-guessed; who believe Americans should trust their lives with their expert opinions.

Take for example the 2002 FDA approval of the ADHD "treatment" Strattera (atomoxetine HCl). Lilly, the maker of Strattera, has heralded the new ADHD "treatment" as "the first and only non-stimulant medication approved by the U.S. Food and Drug Administration." That's right; Strattera is not a stimulant, like other ADHD treatments Adderall and Ritalin. The new Lilly drug is a treatment from the SNRI (selective norepinephrine reuptake inhibitor) class of antidepressants, similar to the popular antidepressant Effexor (venlafoxine HCl). How does Strattera work (the mechanism) in the treatment of ADHD? Well, the simple truth is nobody really knows. The FDA explains the pharmacodynamics this way (in part): "the precise mechanism by which atomoxetine (Strattera) produces its therapeutic effects in Attention-Deficit/ Hyperactivity Disorder (ADHD) *is unknown, but is thought to be* related to.." the chemicals in the brain, blah, blah, blah.[17] (italics mine) In other words, the FDA does not know with any scientific certainty how the drug works, but *thinks* it works a certain way. Lilly is just as clueless about the specific mechanism of its new ADHD drug explaining (in part) *"It is not known precisely* how Strattera reduces ADHD symptoms, but scientists *believe* it works by blocking or slowing reabsorption of norepinephrine.." brain chemicals blah, blah, blah.[18] (italics mine)

Okay, time for a recap. Neither the FDA nor the pharmaceutical giant knows for sure how Strattera treats the alleged mental disorder, and recall from Chapter 4 the 21 words uttered by the psycho-wizards looking into the cause of ADHD: "Finally, after years of clinical research and experience with ADHD, our knowledge about the cause or causes of ADHD remains speculative." In total, nobody knows anything about what exactly is the alleged mental disorder ADHD (except opinions about individual behavior), and nobody knows with certainty how the alleged treatment works. Given that the FDA has approved all of the antidepressants on the market today without any certainty about how the drugs work on the alleged mental illness; it is not surprising that Strattera also would get the agency's stamp of approval. But it is the FDA's failure to include Strattera in the October 2004 list of antidepressants slated to receive "black box" warnings that further diminishes confidence in the agency's belief that its "highly trained scientists" are infallible.

First, though, recall that Strattera hit the news in a big way when the FDA released a December 2004 warning advising health-care professionals about the potential for Strattera to cause severe liver injury. The new labeling warns (in part): "severe liver injury may progress to liver failure resulting in death or the need for a liver transplant in a small percentage of patients."[19] The drug approval agency further explained, "The labeling also notes that the number of actual cases of severe liver injury is unknown because of underreporting of post-marketing adverse events."[20] The FDA reports that the warning was issued because of two known cases of liver injury in a teenager and an adult who had been treated with Strattera. Eli Lilly advises that "post-marketing reports indicate that Strattera can cause liver injury in rare cases, although evidence of liver injury was detected in clinical trials of about 6,000 patients."

Neither Lilly nor the FDA publicly provided any detailed information about the rate of liver injury found during the clinical trials, and beyond the numbers listed above, the 2002 FDA approval letter for Strattera makes no mention of potential liver injury. The 2004 FDA warning issued about Strattera's potential for liver injury is interesting given that the agency apparently was taking the action based on just two reports of liver damage.

Recall that the FDA has received at least 30,000 adverse event reports for the mind-altering Prozac, many of which involve suicide and attempted suicide, and yet it took the drug approval agency 13 years just to place "black box" warnings on it and other antidepressants. If it really is just two cases of liver injury, the Strattera warning seems odd, given the drug agency's liberal attitude toward allowing tens of thousands of adverse reactions for antidepressants. One can only speculate, though, until the FDA and Lilly make public the clinical trial data pertinent to the numbers of patients who experienced the serious liver problems.

But liver injury is not Strattera's only adverse effect. Despite the fact that Strattera is in the SNRI antidepressant class of drugs, it was not until one full year after the public was warned about the increased risk of suicidal and other harmful behaviors associated with antidepressants that the FDA issued a warning for Strattera. The lag time in warning the public about Strattera's "increased risk of suicidal behavior" is of interest in light of the fact that the FDA early on had information about the adverse effects. The insert label for Strattera reveals that the clinical trial data the FDA used to approve the mind-altering drug showed between 2 percent and 5 percent of the patients experienced mood swings, 8 percent experienced irritability and 1 percent had to be discontinued from the trials because of aggression or irritability. Furthermore, in the September 2004 issue of *Pediatrics*, the journal of the American Academy of Pediatrics, a study titled "Aggression, Mania, and Hypomania Induction Associated With Atomoxetine," was published which revealed that 33 percent of the patients reviewed exhibited extreme irritability, aggression, mania or hypomania.[21] These are the same adverse reactions listed for most, if not all, of the antidepressants that landed on the "black box" list.

Finally, though, in September 2005, the FDA requested that Lilly update its Strattera product label to reflect increased suicidal thoughts among children and adolescents. In a press release, the pharmaceutical company explains the action this way (in part): "Lilly submitted to regulatory agencies an analysis of adverse event data from its Strattera clinical trials database that identified a small but statistically significant increased risk of suicidal thoughts among Strattera-treated children and adolescents…"[22] What Lilly found in its review of its clinical trial data was that 0.4 percent of the treated patients, compared to 0 percent of the non-treated, experienced suicidal thoughts. That is four children out of 1,000 who may experience suicidal thoughts. Put another way, if Lilly's figures are correct, and 3 million prescriptions have been written for Strattera, 12,000 children may be affected by these adverse reactions.

Doesn't sound so insignificant at that number but, hey, that's the acceptable risk. There are two questions, though, that come to mind when one considers that the psychiatric, mind-altering drug had been on the market for three years before the FDA acted to warn the public. First, did Lilly turn over all the adverse reaction data to the FDA prior to approval and, if so, how did the "highly trained scientists" at the drug approval agency miss the "statistically significant" increased risk of suicidal thoughts during the 2002 approval process, and then again in 2004 when the antidepressant "black box" list was being considered? Oops! I forgot. The FDA does not believe Americans should have the right to "second-guess" the drug approval decisions made by its "highly trained scientists."

The ever-increasing "warnings" stacking up against GlaxoS-mithKline's, (formerly SmithKline Beecham) antidepressant Paxil (paroxetine HCl) are another example of exactly why Americans cannot and should not depend on the psycho-pharma wizards at the FDA to look out for their best interests. The SSRI antidepressant Paxil was approved by the FDA in 1992 for treatment of depression and certain alleged anxiety disorders. Since its introduction, it has generated tens of billions of dollars in revenues for the British phar-maceutical giant and is considered one of the top three antidepres-sants on the market.

Despite the company's long-held stand that the mind-altering Paxil did not cause suicidal and other harmful behaviors, in 2001 a jury in Cheyenne, Wyo., thought otherwise and found in favor of the relatives of Donald Schell, who three years earlier had taken the drug for just two days when he shot and killed his wife, daughter, granddaughter and then himself. While attorneys for GlaxoSmithKline argued that it was Schell's depression that caused the murderous/suicidal behavior, the jury wasn't buying it and found in favor of Schell's relatives, awarding the family $6.4 million in damages.

What a difference a day makes! At the time of the 2001 Schell trial, the pharmaceutical company's attorneys argued that "there is no evidence linking Paxil to suicide or homicide." Charles F. Preuss, GlaxoSmithKline's lead attorney, said "we believe once the appellate court has a chance to review the scientific evidence, we will prevail."[23] And Preuss further explained, "We do not believe Paxil was responsible for what happened; in fact, extensive clinical studies and more than 70 million patient treatments worldwide since 1991 have shown Paxil to be an effective and generally well-tolerated treatment for depression and other psychiatric disorders."

[24] As usually is the case, the classic psycho-pharma defense of "it was the mental illness that made him do it, not the drug," didn't fly in Wyoming, and it was the company's own internal documents showing GlaxoSmithKline was aware of a small number of people who could become agitated or violent on the drug that apparently won over the jury. And it also appears that what the pharmaceutical company knew and what it made available to the public about its mind-altering drug has caused further problems.

In June 2004, New York State Attorney General Eliot Spitzer brought suit against GlaxoSmithKline alleging the pharmaceutical company had engaged in persistent fraud with respect to Paxil, suppressing results of studies showing the drug was ineffective on children and also that they knew of an increased risk of suicidal behavior. According to Spitzer, *"GSK has engaged in repeated and persistent fraud by misrepresenting, concealing and otherwise failing to disclose to physicians information in its control concerning the safety and efficacy of its antidepressant medication paroxetine HCl ("paroxetine") in treating children and adolescents with Major Depressive Disorder ("MDD")."* [25]

To the layman, what the New York attorney general was alleging was that GlaxoSmithKline knew Paxil was neither safe nor effective in treating depression in the adolescent population and, in fact, "engaged in deceptive, fraudulent and unlawful practices" to push the sale of the drug. Spitzer's complaint is not to be missed, and the following are just a few points he uses to make his case.

- GSK has misrepresented information concerning the safety and efficacy of paroxetine for treating MDD in children and adolescents. GSK has allowed positive information about pediatric use of paroxetine to be disclosed publicly, but has withheld and concealed negative information concerning the safety and efficacy of the drug as treatment for pediatric MDD.

- GSK's studies did not demonstrate that paroxetine is efficacious in treating children and adolescents with MDD.

- Two of the three GSK placebo-controlled studies (377 and 701) failed to show that paroxetine was more effective than placebo or that there was any evidence of efficacy for treating MDD in children and adolescents.

- Study 377 found that "[n]o clinically or statistically significant differences were detected between paroxetine and placebo in either of the [two] primary efficacy variables," or on any of the secondary measures.

- GSK's studies showed the possibility of a link between paroxetine and an increased risk of suicidal thoughts and acts in adolescents. Combined, studies 329, 377 and 701 showed that certain possibly suicide-related behaviors were approximately two times more likely in the paroxetine group than in the placebo group.

- An internal GSK document from 1998 concluded that, in light of the mixed efficacy outcomes from study 329 and the entirely negative results of study 377, GSK's "target" was "t[o] effectively manage the dissemination of these data in order to minimize any potential negative commercial impact."

Clearly, Spitzer had the pharmaceutical giant by the "neurotransmitters," and just two months after Spitzer filed the suit GlaxoSmithKline quietly resolved the matter by agreeing to disclose both positive and negative results about safety and efficacy of its drugs. The company further agreed to pay $2.5 million in fines to the state of New York.

Some punishment, huh? A pharmaceutical company effectively lies about the efficacy of its drug for the treatment of adolescents, gets caught doing so and the punishment consists of being told to do what it should have done to begin with, and then has to cough up a measly $2.5 million in fines. This "agreement" is an insult to the people who may have been harmed by the drug, especially considering that Spitzer made a point of noting that in 2002 alone 900,000 prescriptions for Paxil were written for adolescents, totaling $55 million in revenues for GlaxoSmithKline. Does the old saying "laughing all the way to the bank" come to mind?

But this is just more fuel for the fire that is raging over the FDA's recent policy decision to protect the pharmaceuticals from lawsuits. And, although GlaxoSmithKline slid out of the New York suit with barely a scratch, its top selling Paxil was about to get additional adverse attention.

In October 2004 the FDA announced that Paxil was on the list of antidepressants that would require the new "black box" warnings about the increased risk of suicidal thinking and behavior in children and adolescents; a few months later adults would be added to the list. But Paxil hit the press again when the FDA announced in a December 2005 FDA Public Health Advisory warning that "the FDA has determined that exposure to paroxetine (Paxil) in the first trimester of pregnancy may increase the risk for congenital malformations, particularly cardiac malformations."[26]

Okay, time for a reality check. Paxil may increase suicidal actions and behavior in children and adults, *and* the mind-altering drug also may increase the risk of serious birth defects. Given that it obviously takes a long time (at least a decade) to uncover all of the adverse reactions associated with Paxil and other antidepressants, there's no telling what awful things the "highly trained scientists" may find in the future. GlaxoSmithKline alleges Paxil "treats" depression, something many women may suffer from when they start to put 2 and 2 together. Geesch! One can only wonder how many children were born with cardiac defects in the last decade to women who were being "treated" with Paxil.

An entire book could be written about the ever-increasing number of liability lawsuits being brought against pharmaceutical companies due to alleged harm caused by the psychiatric mind-altering drug products. While it is clear that the FDA believes its drug approval decisions are beyond reproach, information being made public as a result of these legal battles paints a very different picture. The FDA must depend on the drug companies to provide all the positive *and* negative information about the safety and efficacy of a particular drug, and it is not completely clear whether the FDA has been provided all the information needed in the drug approval process or whether it simply ignores it. And, worse still, much to its detriment, it appears that the consuming public is the last to know. Then again, if Dr. Breggin is correct and the FDA only requires that two or three clinical trials support a statistically significant positive response to a drug to prove safety and efficacy, then the information gleaned from the other numerous failed trials doesn't stop the drug from being approved. This FDA standard resembles a try, try, try again approach to drug approval and the public has become the pharmaceutical experimental playground.

But even on a most basic issue, the FDA cannot be counted on. Remember, it is the FDA that refuses to disclose when it became aware of Eli Lilly's "missing" Prozac documents, which most certainly would have a bearing on the FDA's approval of the first of the SSRI antidepressants, Prozac. Why? This request is not above the pay grades of any of the FDA's "highly trained scientists." Either the FDA has the Lilly information, and can document when the information was received, or it doesn't. The American people are not, and should not be treated as, guinea pigs in some vast national drug experiment, only to learn years or decades later that the experiment went terribly wrong for the "statistically significant" few. Until the FDA and pharmaceutical companies can be trusted to provide all the documentation in order to make informed decisions—the good, bad and ugly—those harmed must have an avenue of redress.

In the case of psychotropic drugs, though, it is not a one-sided issue. As has been well-established throughout this book, the legitimacy of the psychiatric diagnosis never is considered, even though the diagnosis must precede the prescribing of psychiatric mind-altering drugs. The psycho-wizards at the APA have never been forced to prove that an objective, confirmable abnormality exists for even a single psychiatric diagnosis. Depression, bi-polar, obsessive-compulsive disorder, anxiety and schizophrenia, to name a few, are alleged mental disorders that are arrived at based on the individual clinician's understanding of a person's behavior, based on criteria (lists of symptoms) listed in the APA's non-scientific psychiatric bible, the *DSM-IV*.

Worse, still, in an apparent attempt to gain legitimacy within the medical community, the deep thinkers on Planet Psycho-pharma persist in misleading the public about the alleged cause(s) of mental disorders by pushing the "chemical imbalance" theory. This theory is not only used as the "believed" cause of the alleged mental abnormality, but is further utilized by the pharmaceutical companies to support the so-called "treatments" that allege to correct, or balance, the theoretical imbalances of the naturally occurring chemicals in the brain.

No one in the scientific, medical or pharmaceutical communities today can measure the levels of any living individual's brain chemicals or know whether they are in or out of balance, nor do they know what the correct chemical levels are for any individual. In fact, a test that measures a living person's brain chemicals does not even exist. And, yet, it is this theory—the chemical imbalance—that has become the modern day mantra of Planet Psycho-pharma to sell mental illness as an abnormality of the brain and the psychiatric mind-altering drugs as the alleged treatments. Tens of millions of Americans have been led to believe they suffer from a measurable brain abnormality and that the psychiatric mind-altering drugs will correct the abnormality. This could not be further from the truth.

Until the psychiatric community is forced to prove that even one of the nearly 400 alleged psychiatric mental disorders is an objective, confirmable abnormality of the brain, the number of American's being subjectively diagnosed as mentally ill and becoming psychiatric drug "users" will continue to increase. And it appears that the FDA is well aware of the explosive increase in mind-altering drugs and also that the now acknowledged adverse effects could prove to be financially painful to the drug makers.

In fact, just weeks after the FDA announced its proposed policy of federal pre-emption, in essence removing the right of the People to sue pharmaceutical companies in state courts, a committee of the drug approval agency met to consider the long-term adverse effects of ADHD "treatments," such as Ritalin, Adderall, Concerta and

Strattera, due to reports of cardiovascular deaths and other related injuries.

The committee shocked the psycho-wizards at the FDA when it recommended that prominent "black box" warnings be added to the labeling of the ADHD drugs. Despite the concerns raised by the committee about the mind-altering ADHD "treatments," panel member, Steven Nissen, MD., a cardiologist at the Cleveland Clinic, said "I have grave concerns about the use of these drugs and grave concerns about the harm they may cause." Regardless of this "grave concern" the FDA apparently intends to ignore the recommendations and follow the same wait and see policy as it took on the antidepressants.[27]

Although the committee voted 8 to 7 to recommend the most serious warnings be added to the ADHD drugs, Dr. Thomas Laughren, director of the Division of Psychiatry Products at the drug approval agency, (one of the "highly trained scientists") said "we don't think anything different needs to be done right now…we think the labeling is adequate."[28] This is perfect. Despite the fact that methylphenidate has been in use since 1955, the high priests of the FDA again appear to be taking the low road, suggesting that the 25 known deaths and dozens of other reported adverse cardiovascular events associated with ADHD drugs are an acceptable risk.

But what has been missed by the public in all the clamor about the potentially harmful effects of ADHD "treatments" is that the cardiovascular events are *NOT* caused by the alleged abnormality ADHD. Rather, what is at issue is that it is the mind-altering "treatments" that are causing the deadly and life-threatening events. This, of course, goes to the very heart of subjective, "speculative" psychiatric diagnosing of the alleged mental illness, ADHD, and every other psychiatric diagnosis.

Until the medical community and policymakers address the lack of science to support any of the psychiatric diagnoses, Americans will continue to be diagnosed with alleged mental abnormalities and the unknowing participants in what can only be described as a mass pharmaceutical clinical trial. It is anyone's guess whose loved one tragically will be counted among those that the psycho-wizards consider the acceptable risk. Americans must decide if they are willing to put their lives in the hands of the "highly trained scientists" whose best diagnosis and "treatment" is based on mere beliefs and speculation.

[1] "FDA Announces New Prescription Drug Information Format to Improve Patient Safety," FDA News, January 18, 2006.

[2] Anna Wilde Mathews, "FDA Plan Would Aid Drug Makers in Liability Suits," *The Wall Street Journal*, January 14, 2006

[3] Marc Kaufman, FDA Tries to Limit Drug Suits in State Courts, *The Washington Post*, January 19, 2006.

[4] Peter Breggin, M.D. and Ginger Ross Breggin: "Talking Back To Prozac: What Doctors Aren't Telling You About Today's Most Controversial Drug," St. Martin's Press, June 1994.

[5] Ibid., Pg-42.

[6] Ibid., Pg-44.

[7] Ibid., Pg-46.

[8] Ibid., pg-47.

[9] Ibid., Pg-47.

[10] Ibid., Pg-47.

[11] Mitchell Zuckoff, "Prozac data was kept from trial, suit says," *The Boston Globe*, June 8, 2000.

[12] Eli Lilly and Company, www.Prozac.com, "How Prozac Can Help: How it Works."

[13] Gurkirpal Singh, M.D., Adjunct Clinical Professor of Medicine, Department of Medicine, Division of Gastroenterology and Hepatology, Stanford University School of Medicine, Testimony, U.S. House of Representatives, Subcommittee on Health of the Committee on Energy and Commerce, February 10, 2005.

[14] Ibid.

[15] Ibid.

[16] Ibid.

[17] Attachment to FDA Approval Letter for NDA 21-411, Strattera (Atomoxetine HC1), pg-1.

[18] Eli Lilly and Company, "Lilly Announces Important Strattera Label Update," September 29, 2005.

[19] FDA Talk Paper, "New Warning for Strattera," December 17, 2004.

[20] Ibid.

[21] Theodore A. Henderson, M.D., PhD., Matrix ADHD Diagnostic Clinic, Neurobehavioral Research, Keith Hartman, M.D., "Aggression, Mania, and Hypomania Induction Associated With Atomoxetine," *Pediatrics* Vol. 114 No. 3, September 2004.

[22] Eli Lilly and Company, "Lilly Announces Important Strattera Label Update," September 29, 2005.

[23] Jeff Swiatek, "Antidepressant Maker GlaxoSmithKline Held Liable in Wrongful-Death Case," *Knight Ridder Tribune Business News* KRTBN, June 7, 2001.

[24] Ibid.

[25] The People of the State of New Yor, by Eliot Spitzer vs. GlaxoSmith Kline, plc., June 2, 2004.

[26] FDA Public Health Advisory "Paroxetine," December 8, 2005.

[27] Gardiner Harris, "Warning Urged on Stimulants Like Ritalin," *The New York Times*, February 9, 2006.

[28] Ibid.

Appendix A:
Books for Further Information

Breggin, P.R. (1991). *Toxic psychiatry: Why therapy, empathy, and love must replace the drugs, electroshock, and biochemical theories of the "new psychiatry."* New York: St. Martin's

Breggin, P.R. (1998). *Talking Back to Ritalin.* Monroe, Maine: Common Courage Press

Breggin, P.R., & Breggin G.R. (1994). *Talking Back to Prozac.* New York: St. Martin's Press.

Valenstein, E.S. (1998). *Blaming the Brain: The truth about drugs and mental health.* New York: Free Press.

Breggin, P.R., & Cohen, David, (1999). *Your Drug May Be Your Problem: How and Why To Stop Taking Psychiatric Medications.* Perseus Books. Reading, Massachusetts.

Breggin, P.R. (2000) *Reclaiming Our Children: A Healing Plan for a Nation In Crisis.* Perseus Books.

Breggin, P.R., *The Ritalin Fact Book: What Your Doctor Won't Tell You About ADHD and Stimulant Drugs.* Perseus Books.

Breggin, P.R. (2001) *The AntiDepressant Fact Book: What Your Doctor Won't Tell You About Prozac, Zoloft, Paxil, Celexa and Luvox.* Perseus Publishing.

Breggin, P.R. (1997) *Brain Disabling Treatments in Psychiatry: Drugs, Electroshock, and The Role of the FDA.* Springer Publishing.

Baughman, Fred A. & Hovey, Craig (2005) *The ADHD Fraud: How Psychiatry Makes "Patients" of Normal Children.* Trafford Publishing.

Moynihan, Ray & Cassels, Alan, (2005). *Selling Sickness: How the World's Biggest Pharmaceutical Companies are Turning Us All Into Patients.* Nation Books.

Dineen, Tana, (1996). *Manufacturing Victims: What the Psychology Industry is Doing to People.* Robert Davies Multimedia Publishing.

Kutchins, Herb & Kirk, Stuart, (1997). *Making Us Crazy: DSM: The Psychiatric Bible and the Creation of Mental Disorders.* The Free Press.

Wiseman, Bruce, (1995) *Psychiatry: The Ultimate Betrayal.* Freedom Publishing.

Eakman, B.K., (1998) *Cloning of the American Mind: Eradicating Morality Through Education.* Huntington House Publishers.

Caplan, Paula, J., (1995) *They Say You're Crazy: How the World's Most Powerful Psychiatrists Decide Who's Normal.* Addison-Wesley Publishing.

Breeding, John, (1996) *The Wildest Colts Make the Best Horses: What to Do When Your Child Is Labeled A Problem by the Schools.* Bright Books, Inc.

Glenmullen, Joseph, (2000) *Prozac Backlash: Overcoming the Dangers of Prozac, Zoloft, Paxil, and Other Antidepressants with Safe, Effective Alternatives.* Touchstone.

Hagan, Margaret, (1997) *Whores of the Court: The Fraud of Psychiatric Testimony and the Rape of American Justice.* Regan Books.

Tracy, Ann Blake, (2001) *Prozac: Panacea or Pandora?* Cassia Publications.

Whitaker, Robert, (2002) *Mad In America: Bad Science, Bad Medicine, And The Enduring Mistreatment of the Mentally Ill.* Perseus Books.

Szasz, Thomas S., (1974) *The Myth of Mental Illness: Foundations of a Theory of Personal Conduct.* (Revised Edition). Harper & Row Publishers.

Appendix B
Useful Internet Websites

www.Breggin.org

www.antidepressantsfacts.com

www.ablechild.org

www.worstpills.org

www.Prozactruth.com

www.mindfreedom.org

www.AHRP.org

www.CCHR.org

www.ADHDfraud.org

www.teenscreen.com

www.ritalindeath.com

www.kidsagainstdrugs.com

www.psychsearch.net

www.nih.gov

www.psych.org

www.fda.gov

www.fightforkids.com

www.blockcenter.com

Index Entries for Psyched Out

G

Gary Cheslek 9
Gender Identity Disorder 26
GlaxoSmithKline 2, 49, 50, 104, 128,
      129, 153, 195, 196, 197, 198
Glenn McIntosh 8
Graham Aldred 2, 16

H

Health Canada 81, 82
Herb Kutchins ix, 32
heroin 24, 66, 68
HHS 79
Homosexuality 25, 26, 32
House Energy and Commerce Sub-
      committee on Oversight and
      Investigations 74

I

If It Runs in Your Family: Depression
      44
IMR Patient Flow Model 2
IMS Health 2, 155
Inhalant Intoxication 29
International Center for Study of Psy-
      chiatry and Psychology 74
International Center for the Study of
      Psychiatry and Psychology 53
Irving Kirsch 54

J

Janssen 52, 153, 154
Jeffrey A. Schaler, Ph.D. 31
Jerry Radke 52
Jim Rosack 16
Johnson & Johnson 72, 153
Jonathan Leo 47
Joseph A. Califano 68
Joseph Glenmullen, M.D. 56

K

Ken Silverstein 52

L

Lawrence Stevens 32
Lexapro 10, 49
Listening to Prozac but Hearing
      Placebo: A Meta Analysis of
      Antidepressant Medication 54
Loren Mosher 34, 43
Loren Mosher, M.D. 34, 43
Luvox 10, 12, 50, 56, 92, 95, 96, 98,
      205
Lynne Rosewater 32

M

Major Depressive Disorder (MDD) 7,
      10, 14, 15, 37
Major Depressive Episode 24
Making Us Crazy: The Psychiatric
      Bible and the Creation of Men-
      tal Disorders 32
Margaret Hagen 31
Mark Miller 8
Mark Taylor 12
Masochistic Personality Disorder 32
Mathematics Disorder 27
McNeil Pharmaceuticals 72
MDD 7, 10, 14, 15, 37, 105, 196, 197
Medco Health Solutions 83, 155
Medicines and Healthcare products
      Regulatory Agency 6
methadone 24, 66
Methylphenidate 23, 65, 66, 67, 69,
      72, 77, 78, 79, 80, 83, 201
methylphenidate HCl 72, 78
mirtazapine 48, 49

N

NAMI 50, 51, 52, 152, 180
National Institute of Mental Health
      (NIMH) 35
New Yorker magazine 33
Nicotine Dependence 30
Nicotine Withdrawal 30
NIH 75, 77, 81

Printed in the United States
120448LV00003B/2/A